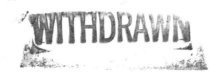

Horses' Injuries

by the same author

*

COMMON-SENSE THERAPY FOR HORSES' INJURIES

HORSES' INJURIES

Common-sense Therapy of Muscles and Joints for the Layman

CHARLES L. STRONG

MVO, MCSP

With a Foreword by
Admiral of the Fleet the Earl Mountbatten of Burma, K.G.

ARCO PUBLISHING COMPANY, INC.
New York

Published 1973 by Arco Publishing Company, Inc.
219 Park Avenue South, New York, N.Y. 10003

Copyright © 1967 by Charles L. Strong

Library of Congress Catalog Card Number 72-97583
ISBN 0-668-02959-5

Printed in Great Britain

(

Contents

Illustrations

Illustrations

Foreword

BY ADMIRAL OF THE FLEET THE EARL MOUNTBATTEN OF BURMA, K.G.

When I was Captain of the Bluejackets Polo Team, which represented the Royal Navy in the Inter-Regimental Tournaments before the war, we all relied upon Mr. Charles Strong's treatment to repair the inevitable damage most polo players sustain from collisions, accidents and falls during the course of a season.

In 1939 I asked him the question which triggered-off the new treatment he has developed for horses—'Since you can cure the polo players so quickly, when they have injuries, why don't you use your same treatment to cure their polo ponies?'

Mr. Strong immediately tried his treatment with instant and gratifying success, but then the war intervened and nothing more could be done until he had been demobilized and was back in practice.

I started playing polo again after the war and renewed my request that he should treat my ponies as well as myself. He did this and extended his treatment to racehorses, hunters and other horses and animals with sensational success.

I am a confirmed believer in his treatment for lameness in horses as I have abundant proof of the seemingly miraculous cures he has been able to achieve with my own ponies.

I am, therefore, delighted to recommend this book very strongly to anyone who is interested in curing lameness in horses.

Mountbatten of Burma,
A.F.

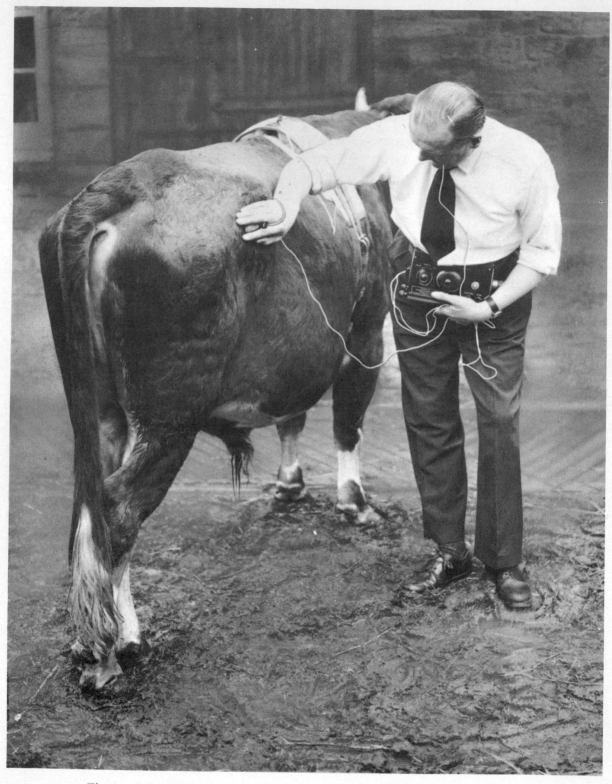

Fig. 1.   A Guernsey bull being treated for a sprain of Rt. stifle joint. Treatment was completed successfully and the animal resumed normal duties within a fortnight of the first treatment

Preface

When reviewing my book *Common Sense Therapy for Horses' Injuries* Colonel Colin Davy said that an effort should be made to produce a version more easily understood by laymen.

Since then nine years have passed and during that time many laymen have passed similar opinions, pointing out that if they could follow the main principles easily they would be able to co-operate to the full when treatment was applied. I would go further than this and say there is no reason at all why the experienced horse layman should not apply the treatment himself, provided the case has been previously diagnosed by a veterinary surgeon and the treatment is under the latter's supervision.*

If the method is to become common practice, and it is applied at the right time, there are insufficient properly trained people to cope with the number of cases, so perforce it will fall to the lot of the suitable layman, or laywoman, to carry out the treatment.

Having said this I must point out that it is not just a matter of switching on and switching off. There is a definite technique and an art to the whole process. However, two to three months daily practice should produce reasonable proficiency and, in fact, this is just what is happening in many parts of the world.

As the method of treatment is a joint effort between the veterinary surgeon prescribing or carrying out the treatment, and the people responsible for the stable management and the prescribed exercise, I endeavoured to give a simplified version. This proved difficult as one wanted to explain technicalities in too much detail. It therefore had to be edited by a knowledgeable horse layman.

As he was the first to say this was necessary, who better to do the job than Colonel Davy himself? I was delighted when he consented. He has laboured indefatigably with manuscript and proof. Descriptions which I thought clear and simple were, I fear, unintelligible until edited by him.

I also owe gratitude to Dr. A. C. Fraser, PH.D., B.V.SC., M.R.C.V.S. for his interest and ever courteous advice on matters relating to horses in general and for reporting in the *Veterinary Record* (February 4th 1961, Vol. 73, No. 5, pp. 94–100) the results of one hundred cases of lameness or defective action he observed treated by me. It was not

* Obligatory under Veterinary Surgeon's Act 1948.

surprising to find that eighty-eight were cured. This 88 per cent of cures might have been increased had some of the twelve failures come under treatment earlier.

Though never my intention to produce special apparatus, that available was not the most suitable to horses or to the treatment of very recent injury, so one was obliged to design an appropriate instrument. This has passed through many stages of development. The present instrument, the 'SEVA', has evolved and is the ideal instrument. So my thanks are due to the manufacturers, Messrs. Transeva, Jordans Farm, Forest Green, Dorking, Surrey, England, and for their permission to publish certain photographs; to the artist Mr. D. L. Travis for his care over the drawings; to my publishers for their kindness and patience.

Lastly, my undying gratitude to Admiral of the Fleet the Earl Mountbatten of Burma, K.G. for the original idea, in 1939, of applying this treatment to horses and other animals. His unstinted encouragement and guidance over a great number of years, without which neither the treatment itself, this book, nor *Common Sense Therapy for Horses' Injuries* would have seen light of day, and to whom my grateful thanks for the Forewords to both.

I have not quoted from other works on this subject relative to horses, as they do not exist, and it seems better to write from personal experience.

If this method of treatment is a contribution to veterinary science then I am more than satisfied.

C. L. Strong,
73 Portland Place,
London, W.1.

CHAPTER I

Introduction

As far as strain, sprain and bruising are concerned, the treatment least likely to bring relief is over-rest, especially if enforced during the early stages of these injuries. Yet it is the usual procedure despite the fact that it contributes to disability and not to its relief; and so from this mistaken idea that rest is 'Nature's Method' a great number of horses, even valuable horses, and other animals are lost to the purpose for which they were required.

It will, of course, be argued that painful movement is 'Nature's call for rest'. It would be instructive to know when Nature proclaimed this and where it is recorded. However, even if true, it surely means *rest only throughout that range of movement which is painful*.

In all injuries to muscles and joints there is a range of movement, either in the affected joint or in the joints above or below the affected joint and in the muscles, which is painless. This painless movement might be small but, nevertheless, it is present. If Nature intended pain to be answered by rest throughout the full range of movement it would have made the full range of movement painful.

As it has not done so it is safe, and scientifically proved not only safe but beneficial, to assume that Nature intended the part to be moved throughout the painless range of movement.

If this is done—painlessly—from the earliest possible moment the rate of recovery is not only greater but more complete than by any other form of treatment.

If Nature were to make any proclamation it would surely be 'intensive movement throughout the painless range of movement immediately following the injury and subsequently.'

It has been known for a very long time that repair of damaged tissue depends upon a good circulation of blood, but the word 'circulation' means a circulatory movement.

To bring more blood to a part, such as by the application of heat in any of its various forms, or blistering, etc., is to move blood in one direction only. It is not increasing the true circulation. In fact, heat, blistering, etc., can bring so much blood to the part that the subsequent congestion actually reduces the true circulation.

Therefore, if there is such a thing as 'Nature's requirement' it is for painless movement and a good circulation. It is hoped in the following pages to prove to the layman that to enforce rest accompanied by any of the above applications is to retard repair and impede the animal's recovery.

It will again be argued that some cases when so treated do recover. Undoubtedly this is so, but it can never be said that the recovery was 'because of', it should be 'despite'. The recovery would most certainly have been quicker and the period of pain reduced if not so treated.

The subject of the treatment of strain, sprain and bruising as it affects the horse, and in fact any animal, is fascinating and of great importance, and when studied and treated scientifically results are obtained which can only be described as brilliant compared with the usual results which are so often a great disappointment. These disappointments are so frequent that the conditions, as far as animals are concerned, are looked upon as incurable.

Not only this, but the difficulty of diagnosing the precise location of a muscular injury was at times very speculative. This to a very great extent has been eliminated, and in the vast majority of cases a precise 'pin-pointing' of the injured part can be made.

This affects not only the individual horse but the far-reaching effects can be of serious concern to breeding of racehorses in general. One has only to consider the injury of a potential Derby winner. Because of a trivial injury he may never have a chance to prove himself on the racecourse. What a loss it would have been to breeding throughout the whole world if Hyperion or Nearco had never been able to prove themselves, and so had been lost to breeding. How many other horses potentially as great, or greater, have been lost for this reason?

Impressed with these facts, the author started the serious study of these injuries to horses; this has been given in full in *Common Sense Therapy for Horses' Injuries*. It is for those who require a fuller explanation than this book provides.

This method of treatment has proved to be, as in the case of humans, in both early and late cases of strain, sprain and bruising, far superior in its results and much quicker in promoting complete recovery than any other method at present in use.

Unfortunately, the faradic current which is used to produce Rhythmic Muscular Contractions is usually looked upon, *even by some who should know better*, only as a means of increasing muscle bulk.

There are several precise techniques for the application of the faradic current, all for different purposes, and each requires a final current of certain characteristics, and Rhythmic Muscular Contractions adds one more.

This is why the author at the outset was faced not only with producing a particular technique, but also an apparatus producing a particular type of faradic current for that technique. It is, therefore, quite *wrong* to class this treatment under the general and vague heading of 'Faradism' as this term gives no indication of what type of faradism and what technique.

Introduction

To those people who look upon it as a means of increasing muscle bulk only, it is quite illogical to apply faradism for an injury to a horse which is fully 'muscled-up' and ready for racing. So no wonder they say 'What can faradism do in this case?' The answer is, of course, 'By using a particular type of faradic current to produce Rhythmic Muscular Contractions the condition will be treated on sound scientific lines and the possibility of restoring full function is greatly enhanced.' Morever, this will, in all probability, be accomplished before muscle wasting and general loss of condition in the horse can take place.

Even in those late cases where muscle wasting has already taken place: relieve the pain by Rhythmic Muscular Contractions and, in consequence, painless exercise of a suitable type will restore the muscle bulk.

It must surely have been with the people who consider the faradic current as a muscle builder only in his mind, when one of the world's most eminent medical practitioners of physical medicine said, in effect, 'The person who knows one technique and one technique only stamps himself as unfit to use the faradic apparatus at all.'

To these should be added 'All those operators of this apparatus who require rubber gloves to protect themselves from the sensation of the current, as it stamps them as not having mastered the technique.' Correctly applied the operator cannot feel the current at all.

The techniques of applying the faradic current are several and diverse. In this book we are concerned with one technique only, i.e. Rhythmic Muscular Contractions, the apparatus for that technique, and to explain its indications and use to the layman.

The object of this book, therefore, is to present to the layman who may be called upon by the veterinarian to give treatment, the principles and technique of the treatment of strain, sprain and bruising by the method of Rhythmic Muscular Contractions.

The restoration of muscle function is of the utmost importance after injuries of every degree, yet when a joint is injured nearly every other component part receives attention, but the muscle condition passes all too often almost unnoticed.

The 'chronic' sprained joint is often regarded as the natural result of an injury and only to be expected, whereas in reality the disability is mostly mechanical, due to the neglected muscular condition occurring at the time of the original injury.

It is the injuries to the deep and superficial flexor tendons, the check and suspensory ligaments of the forelegs, which account for the greatest loss in horses used for fast work.

Injuries to these tendons are not easy to deal with, but much progress has been made. It is, as yet, too early to say 'The answer has been found.' Injuries to the suspensory ligaments are considerably less formidable propositions.

But running the frequency of the above injuries very close are injuries to horses' backs. These often go undetected and the horse is called 'a rogue', or, has 'gone sour', 'lost form', when, in fact, he has a painful condition of back which may show only towards the end of a race or when jumping.

Introduction

Although Rhythmic Muscular Contractions are produced by means of an electrical current, it must be emphasized that no virtue of curative power whatever is claimed from the use of the electricity *per se*. The electrical current is used merely to produce muscular contraction and relaxation, with its attendant chemical and circulatory changes. If there was a means other than electrical to produce the same muscular contractions and relaxations the results would be equally satisfactory.

To obtain a clear conception of the results of treatment by Rhythmic Muscular Contractions it is necessary to discuss briefly the main underlying anatomical, physiological and pathological principles which govern the structure of a joint in health and as a result of injury.

CHAPTER II

A General Description of Muscles and their Function

When considering the stimulation of muscle by electrical means for the treatment of sprain, strain and bruising in horses, it is not essential for the layman to have an extensive knowledge of the muscles and how they are composed, but some idea of the machinery which makes a joint work and of what that machinery consists is an advantage.

Muscle is made up of various structures, and what makes it different from all other body tissues are the fibres which develop the muscular contraction, which causes the movements of the joints they govern.

The properties of muscles in general are:

1. Elasticity—the ability to stretch.
2. Contractility—the ability to contract and shorten.
3. Irritability—sensitiveness.
4. Tone—a healthy liveliness and alertness.

1. **Elasticity** is the ability of a muscle to return to its original shape after its natural action of contracting. The connective tissue which surrounds the muscle fibres, binding them together and giving them strength, is of an elastic nature and provides the muscle's elasticity.

As will be seen from Figure 2 voluntary muscle is composed of bundles of fibres, each individual fibre being surrounded by a sheath of elastic connective tissue. These fibres are collected into bundles and these bundles are enclosed in another sheath of connective tissue. These sheaths are of great importance when considering injury as they are elastic and contain vast numbers of lymphatic vessels. (See Fig. 2).

Muscles are of varying shapes and sizes, each for its own particular purpose. Those having a simple task—such as the muscle which extends the fetlock joint—are simple, long and narrow. (See Fig. 3).

Other muscles having more complicated jobs are more complex in formation. The

19

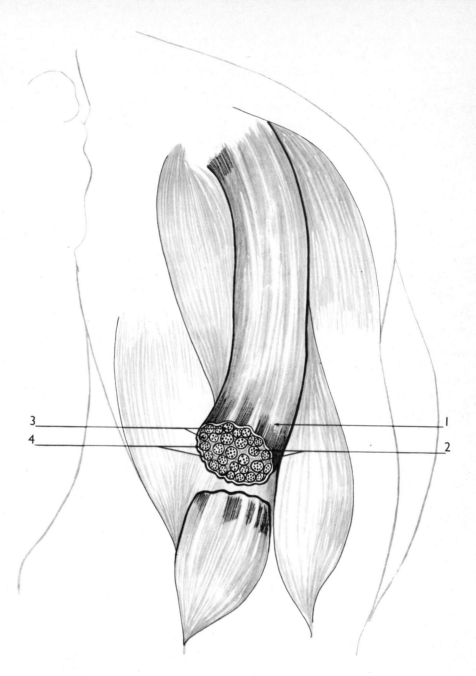

Fig. 2. **Muscle cut across to show cross-section** (*Drawing diagrammatic*)
1. Muscle, 2. Individual muscle fibres collected into bundles and
3. Enclosed in connective tissue sheath, 4. Sheath of whole muscle
These sheaths are made of elastic connective tissue

latissimus dorsi, for instance, has a multitude of actions: (1) Drawing the forelimb backwards and upwards. (2) Flexing the shoulder. (3) When the forelimb is firmly on the ground, drawing the horse's body forward. In consequence it is large, flat and fan-shaped. (See Fig. 4).

Throughout the body each skeletal muscle starts anchored to a fixed point on bone, known as the origin. The other end of the muscle is attached to another bone, beyond the joint over which the muscle has to work, and is called the insertion. These attachments are made of non-elastic tissue, known as tendon. Their attachment to bone is somewhat like seaweed growing into rock. (see Fig. 5).

The elasticity of muscle structure enables a muscle, when fit or in 'tone', to respond instantly to an impulse calling for contraction. In strained or wasted muscles this elasticity or willingness to respond is lost or diminished, like the elastic in a pair of old garters. The elastic strands are unable to contract in harmony with the others of the group, resulting in mechanical inefficiency. The stretchability of a muscle comes from the connective tissue sheaths of the fibres, bundles of fibres, and the sheath of the muscle as a whole, and not from the muscle fibre itself.

The elasticity of the actual muscle fibre, however, must not be likened to that of the sheaths or india-rubber. India-rubber has to be pulled out by a force before it contracts on being released. Muscle fibre in a state of tension contracts on its own accord, and at rest relaxes to the full length required by the position of the joint. So, in fact, the action of the actual muscle fibre is the exact opposite of india-rubber.

2. **Contractility.** This means the ability of a muscle to contract and shorten on the application of a stimulus, such as a message from the nervous system. On the cessation of the stimulus the muscle relaxes.

This process of contraction produces an expenditure of energy, the formation of lactic acid, oxygenation of carbo-hydrates and fats, the consumption of oxygen, and the freeing of carbon-dioxide.

These waste products are produced in the muscles as the result of its activities, and they are removed quickly by the circulation of blood through the muscles. These waste products, if not quickly removed, would inhibit the muscle and interfere with its capacity to contract and relax.

As the blood circulation through a muscle is increased by contraction and relaxation it follows that in wasted, injured or unhealthy muscles the amount of blood circulating is reduced.

It must be remembered that the process of contraction and relaxation is not instantaneous: there is a time factor and, however small this may be, it is slowed down in muscles which have lost their liveliness by injury or become wasted from other causes. Further, it is easy to understand that any slowing-down of muscular efficiency in a single muscle or a group of muscles must interfere with others co-ordinated with it. So,

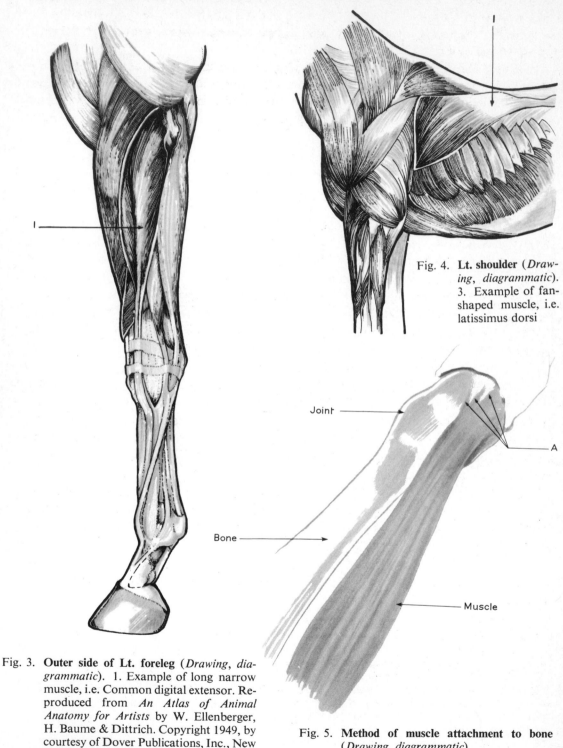

Fig. 4. **Lt. shoulder** (*Drawing, diagrammatic*). 3. Example of fan-shaped muscle, i.e. latissimus dorsi

Joint

Bone

Muscle

A

Fig. 3. **Outer side of Lt. foreleg** (*Drawing, diagrammatic*). 1. Example of long narrow muscle, i.e. Common digital extensor. Reproduced from *An Atlas of Animal Anatomy for Artists* by W. Ellenberger, H. Baume & Dittrich. Copyright 1949, by courtesy of Dover Publications, Inc., New York 14, N.Y.

Fig. 5. **Method of muscle attachment to bone** (*Drawing, diagrammatic*). A. Insertion of muscle

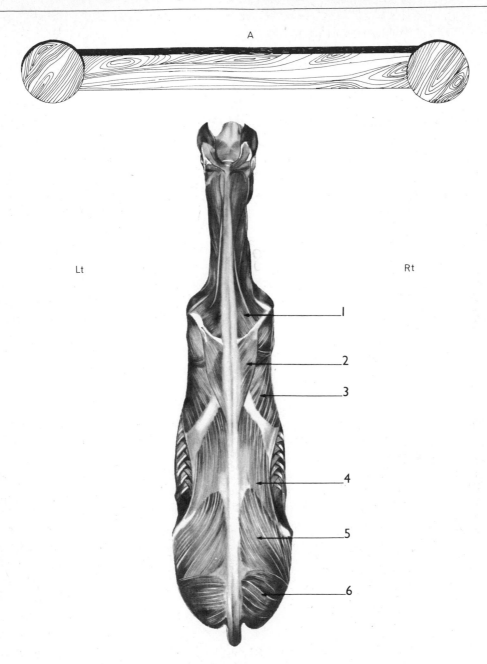

Fig. 6. **Main muscles of back** (*Drawing, diagrammatic*). 1. Trapezius cervicis, 2. Trapezius thorasis, 3. Latissimus dorsi, 4. Longissimus dorsi, 5. Glutius medius, 6. Glutius maximus. If the muscles, or even one muscle, on the right side of the spine are injured, or working less efficiently than those on the left side, when the horse attempts to lift his fore-end to jump the obstacle at 'A' he will swerve to the left owing to the muscles of this side being stronger, or working more efficiently. Reproduced from *An Atlas of Animal Anatomy for Artists* by W. Ellenberger, H. Baume & Dittrich. Copyright 1949, by courtesy of Dover Publications, Inc., New York 14, N.Y.

if a muscle or a group of muscles on one side of a horse's back is even slightly injured it will mean uneven action, as those on one side of the back are not co-ordinated properly with the muscles on the other.

This can account for a horse developing a tendency to jump to one side, or going better on a right-handed than on a left-handed course, and vice versa. (See Fig. 6).

3. **Irritability.** This means that quality in living muscle which responds READILY to a stimulus.

The result of stimulation to a muscle is to produce a state of contraction, and on the removal or cessation of the stimulus the muscle relaxes. This reaction depends on the sensitivity of the muscle and nerves. In muscles wasted, or in those which have lost their liveliness through injury or other causes, the sensitivity is lessened. They are slower to contract and slower to relax.

When muscles, wasted and insensitive through injury, are being treated by electrical stimulation, it is important that the muscles are allowed to relax completely before renewing the stimulus to obtain further contraction. Otherwise they get tired and treatment is useless. The same effect will be got by making the contractions follow too quickly one after the other, or by giving more than about ten consecutive contractions to any one muscle.

The object of treatment is to restore the muscle's sensitivity and liveliness by stimulating it to work in its NATURAL WAY, thereby restoring the circulation and the elimination of waste products.

4. **Muscle Tone.** When a muscle's elasticity, contractility and irritability (or sensitiveness) are normal it may be said to be in 'good tone'. This may be described as a muscle's fitness to respond quickly to a message from the nervous system.

A healthy and really fit muscle is normally in a state of slight continued contraction or semi-tension. This tension is found in horses 'wound-up' to a high state of physical fitness, and this state is recognized by people experienced in judging a horse's state of fitness by running a hand along its muscles. This tension or semi-tension of the muscles is of immense importance in horses wound-up to do fast work, for the muscular responses of a half-fit horse, whose muscles lack 'tone', will not be quick enough to prevent a joint being damaged by the strain of some misadventure at high speed. This tension can be likened to that of a fully wound spring which is always ready to leap into action.

This state of 'tone' is essential to the efficient action of all muscles. Its loss or diminution after even a slight injury is very serious. Furthermore, if an injured muscle does not recover quickly, wasting will follow bringing further complications. It is the elastic connective tissue which, when a muscle is fit, assists in producing immediate reaction to a sudden demand of a muscle's willingness to contract. In an injured muscle there is a feeling of less than normal elasticity (or tension) when examined in a state of relaxation.

24

MUSCLE ACTION

By muscle action is meant the complete sequence from the first stimulus which begins to contract the muscle or group of muscles, making them broaden and shorten, until the movement is finished and the muscle relaxes and lengthens. It also means the action of the opposing muscle, or group of muscles, which give way and relax in relation to its opposite number's contraction. When a person contracts strongly his biceps muscle (in the arm) the opposing muscle along the back of the arm, from elbow to shoulder (triceps), stretches and relaxes to allow the elbow to bend. (See Fig. 7).

This process of muscle action is so marvellously correlated that a muscle can contract throughout its whole range or with only a small part of it. And in the exact proportion of the one contracting the opposing one gives way no matter how fast the movements are carried out.

When muscles act to produce movement a great expenditure of energy results. This is replaced by the oxygen and nutrition brought by the arterial blood to the muscle by its very own contraction. It is estimated that a muscle in action requires six times more blood than when at rest.

The main claim for treatment by Rhythmic Muscular Contractions carried out by electrical stimulation is the increase of circulation to the muscles and NEIGHBOURING TISSUES, restoring their 'tone' and bringing them back to full healthy efficiency again.

CIRCULATION OF THE BLOOD

The circulation of the blood is carried out by three systems: 1. the arteries, 2. the veins and, 3. the lymphatics.

1. **The arteries** are muscular tubes which carry the blood, laden with oxygen and other nutritive contents, from one side of the heart TO the tissues—and as far as this book is concerned, chiefly to the muscles, tendons, ligaments and all other soft tissues in and around muscles, joints as well as to bone—and here it gives up its oxygen and the other nutritive contents to these structures, to make good the wear and tear and the expended energy. (See Fig. 8).

2. **The veins** arise in the tissues and are tubes similar to the arteries but much less muscular and, unlike the arteries, are fitted with valves so that the blood can flow in one direction only. The veins collect part of the blood, now darker in colour, it having given up its oxygen, etc., and having collected waste products FROM the tissues, and returns it TO the heart. This dark-coloured blood is then pushed, by the heart, to the lungs where it picks up fresh oxygen and, in consequence, changes to bright red, and is returned to the heart for the start of the journey to the tissues once more. (See Fig. 8 and 9).

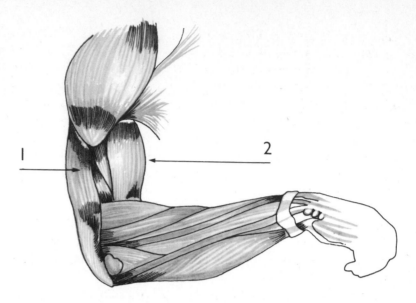

Fig. 7. **Rt. Human arm** (*Drawing, diagrammatic*). 1. Triceps, 2. Biceps. As biceps contracts, the opposing muscle—triceps—must give way to exactly the same extent as biceps contracts to enable movement to take place in the elbow joint.

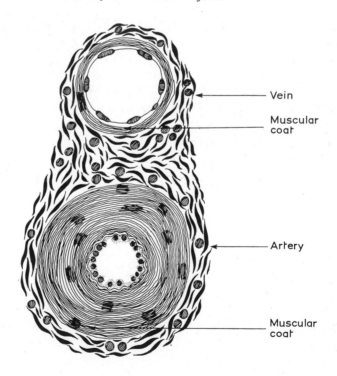

Fig. 8. **Cross section of a vein and an artery.** To show the greater muscular coat of the artery. (*Drawing, diagrammatic*)

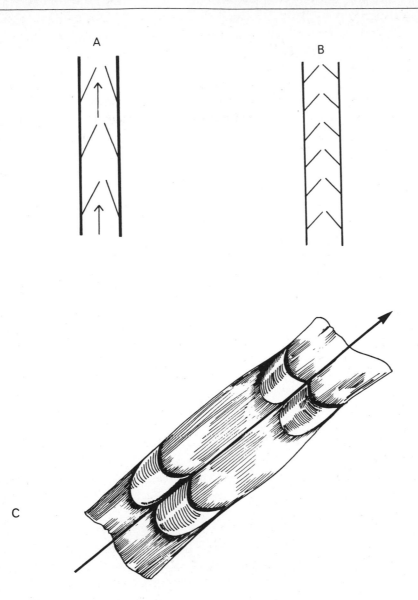

Fig. 9. A. **Longitudinal section of a vein**
B. **Similar section of a lymphatic vessel.** To show the thinner wall and more numerous valves of the lymphatic.
C. **The cup-like construction of the valves which allow the fluid contents of both the vein and lymph vessel to flow in one direction only.** When the fluid contents of these vessels attempt to flow in a direction opposite to that of the arrow the valves open and stop the backward flow of the fluid. (*Drawing, diagrammatic*)

27

3. **The lymphatics** arise in the tissues and in structure are like thin-wall veins. They are provided with numerous valves which, like those of the veins, allow the fluid contents of these vessels to flow in one direction only. They carry FROM the tissues that watery part of the blood known as lymph. (See Fig. 9).

The lymphatic vessels pass to the abdomen, form into a large sac, and here the lymph collects the nutriment from the digestive system. The now nutritive-laden lymph—having changed its colour to a milky-white—is emptied into a vein and mixes with the dark-coloured blood, and it is then taken to the heart, and so on to the lungs and back to the heart, to be introduced once more into the arteries for distribution to the tissues according to their needs. So the nutriment gained from the digestive system, and the oxygen from the lungs, reaches the tissues.

And so the circulation goes on. It must be constantly kept in mind that the word 'circulation' means the full activity of these *three* systems. To bring more blood to a part by means of applying heat, etc., locally, without equally stimulating the venous and lymphatic return may produce such a congestion, especially in the denser tissues, such as tendons, that it will actually clog and reduce the local circulation considerably. This is detrimental to the repair of injured tissue.

MUSCLE NUTRITION AND CIRCULATION

It is estimated that muscles at work require at least six times more blood than when at rest. But the heart is not selective in its distribution of blood. It pumps out into the arteries only a certain amount of blood at each beat and at a certain pressure, and this goes out to all parts of the body.

The tissues requiring most, at a particular moment, make their own arrangements to take more from the arteries. And in the case of muscles when they require more blood for the job they have on hand they fend for themselves. In other words, they create their own method of stepping-up their own *circulation*. A muscle cannot increase the blood supply to itself without automatically increasing the return by means of the veins and lymphatics.

The main artery leaving the heart is very large; it divides and sub-divides, and the branches from the sub-divisions gradually reduce in size as they reach the tissues. On arrival at the muscles they are very small hair-like tubes—now called capillaries. These capillaries are arranged in the muscles in such a manner that at each muscular contraction, and in accordance to the degree of contraction, they become twisted and blood is squeezed from them into the actual muscle fibre, and so the muscle as a whole receives oxygen- and nutritive-laden blood in just the right quantity and at just the right moment when it is most needed for the muscle's well-being.

So the more work the muscles do the more blood is squeezed into them from the capillaries, and the less work they do the less blood is forced into them.

28

Now the more work the muscles do the more waste products are formed and if these are not got rid of quickly they will inhibit the muscle and so reduce its efficiency.

In addition to the waste products produced by the muscular contraction, there is the increased amount of fluid present owing to the increase of arterial blood in the muscle and this, too, must be got rid of, otherwise the part will become engorged and congested with stagnant, de-oxygenated, waste-product-laden blood which, by this time, is also denuded of any nutritive content.

But in the normal uninjured condition this possible congestion is taken care of, chiefly by two methods:

1.   Every time a muscle contracts it compresses the veins and lymphatic vessels in the immediate locality and, owing to the arrangement of the valves in these vessels, this pressure pushes away their contents. So according to the frequency and degree of muscular contraction the venous and lymph flow from the part is stimulated. (See Fig. 10).

2.   The veins and lymphatic vessels are elastic, in the india-rubber sense. As a joint moves in one direction they become stretched, and by the opposite movement of the joint they reduce in length. This movement, again due to the arrangement of the valves, helps to push away the contents of the veins and lymphatics. (See Fig. 11).

So by muscular contraction and relaxation and the movements of the joints caused by the muscular activity, not only is fresh blood brought to the part by the arteries, but the venous and lymphatic flow is equally stimulated, and in the correct proportions relative to one another.

By this activity not only is fresh blood brought to and the used blood pushed away from the actual muscles but also TO and FROM all the SURROUNDING TISSUES.

This is made very apparent by an X-ray photograph of bones which have been in plaster of Paris for some time and therefore deprived of the circulation created by the activity of the surrounding muscles and joints. The bones lose their density (show a rarefied condition) because the bone has been deprived of its normal nutriment.

From this it can easily be understood that muscles which are wasted or have lost their 'tone', and therefore are not working properly, cannot get the nutrition they require for their own maintenance and the circulation to *all the surrounding structures is decreased.*

Returning to the stimulating effect of muscular action on the venous and lymphatic return, and the lack of stimulation of these two systems producing a congestion when the muscles are not working, is well illustrated by the so-called 'Monday morning filling' of a horse's legs after the horse has been stood-in over the week-end. During this period the legs are deprived of the pumping action of the muscles in the upper part

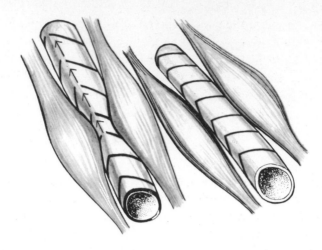

Fig. 10. At each contraction of the surrounding muscles the veins and lymph vessels are compressed and their contents are thereby pushed away in the direction of the arrow. (*Drawing, diagrammatic*)

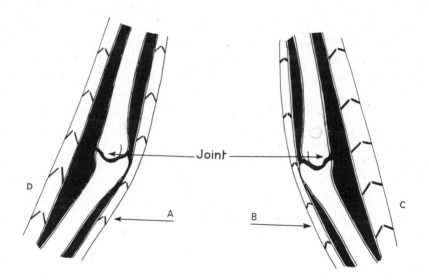

Fig. 11. The stretching and shortening of the veins and lymph vessels by the movement of joints, created by muscular contraction, also increase the flow of their contents, in one direction. So not only is the flow of the contents of the veins and lymphatics increased by muscular contraction, but also by the movement of joints created by the muscular activity. (*Drawing, diagrammatic*)

of the legs and so the lymph and venous blood, aided by gravity, collect and stagnate in the lower part.

The muscular activity and the movements of the joints, so caused on the horse being exercised, quickly pumps this away. This, alone, emphasizes the importance of maintaining muscular activity in the upper part of a leg when the lower part is injured if stagnation of fluids is to be avoided and a healthy circulation maintained, upon which repair of injury is totally dependent.

CONNECTIVE TISSUE

As has been explained, the muscles are sheathed in various ways by elastic connective tissue; the muscle fibres and the bundles of fibres are bound together by elastic connective tissue. The tendons which anchor the muscles at either end to bone are made of non-elastic connective tissue.

There are, however, three different types of connective tissue: A. Areolar tissue, B. Fibrous connective tissue, and C. Elastic connective tissue.

A.   **Areolar Tissue** is a soft loose tissue containing a network of inter-communicating spaces. It possesses great tenacity and elasticity. It is abundantly distributed throughout the body, in fact there is no part without it. Its function must be borne in mind; whilst acting as a supporting bedding between the muscles, blood-vessels, lymphatics, nerves, and all deep-seated structures, it fills up the crevices and spaces. This tissue contains a small amount of lymph-like fluid to keep it moist and supple, and a lack of this fluid may contribute to the creaking and cracking sound which takes place during the action of certain joints in certain conditions. This should not be confused with or mistaken for osteo-arthritis. Lymph and blood escaping from injured vessels can travel a great distance through this tissue.

B.   **Fibrous Connective Tissue** is different from areolar tissue. It is very strong and pliant. It is not elastic, but in certain circumstances it may have an amount of 'give'. Ligaments and tendons requiring great strength are made of it. It has a POOR BLOOD SUPPLY but is WELL ENDOWED with LYMPHATIC VESSELS.

C.   **Elastic Connective Tissue.** The main characteristic is elasticity. For the main part it is used in the make-up of powerful ligaments in the horse's neck and the suspensory ligaments which support the fetlock joints. Like fibrous tissue it has a POOR BLOOD SUPPLY but is WELL ENDOWED with LYMPHATIC VESSELS.

The other tissues which are of concern from an injury point of view are: A. Adipose or fatty tissue, B. Synovial membrane, and C. Cartilage.

31

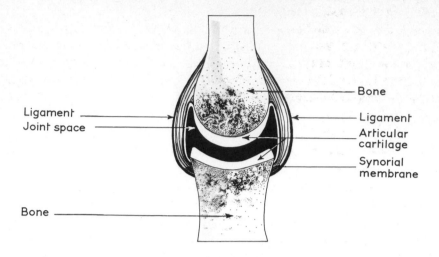

Fig. 12. Longitudinal section of a joint, showing component parts. (*Drawing, diagrammatic*)

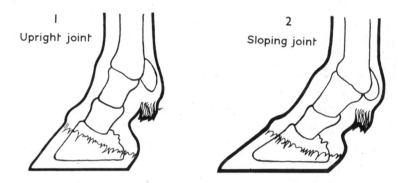

Fig. 13. 1. **An upright pastern**, 2. **A sloping pastern** (*Drawing, diagrammatic*). The joints of the upright pastern will receive a much greater buffeting than those of the sloping pastern, especially when the horse gallops on hard ground.

A.   **Adipose or fatty tissue** is widespread throughout the body. Its presence is important in the neighbourhood of joints to fill up what otherwise would be air-spaces between working parts. It has blood vessels and lymphatics.

B.   **Synovial membrane.** A pliable sheet-like tissue, which secretes a special fluid for lubricating purposes (joint oil). It oils the working surfaces of joints, and grooves in which tendons work, and the opposed surfaces of bursal sacs (these are shock-absorbers between muscles and tendons, skin and harder tissue). In joints, synovial membrane lines the joint cavity. (See Fig. 12).

C. **Cartilage.** As far as joints are concerned this is a firm, tough, but at the same time elastic substance. It forms the ends of bones and, owing to its elastic springiness, acts as a buffer to joints, absorbing shocks. Therefore, the cartilage covering the ends of the bones which form the fetlock joint get a great deal more buffeting in an upright than in a sloping joint. (See Fig. 13).

There is also another type of cartilage—white fibro-cartilage. This forms the discs or flat pads between the vertibrae.

The surface of joint cartilage is moist and slippery on account of the joint oil (synovial fluid); but it also lubricates itself by the worn-off cells caused by friction, these are replaced by those from a deeper layer. So the more a joint is used, the more cells are removed and supply more lubricant.

CHAPTER III

Injury and its immediate effects

When considering the treatment of injury to muscles and OTHER JOINT STRUC-
TURES it is important to understand the changes which take place in these tissues
when they are injured.

Oedema (Filling)

All the tissues of the body are bathed in lymph which exudes from the blood vessels.
There are many causes for an excessive exudation of lymph, but when the tissues are
injured they become saturated with it far beyond the normal; the condition is called
oedema and by the layman often referred to as 'filling'.

The over-saturation of the tissues causes swelling and thus stretches it. The stronger
denser tissues resist the stretching, but the loose, soft areolar tissue does not do so.

Extravasation of Blood

As the result of injury, and according to the severity of the injury, blood is poured
out from the torn arteries, capillaries, veins and lymph from the lymphatic vessels into
the surrounding tissues. This escape of blood undergoes certain changes in the course
of time and ultimately becomes absorbed. During this process its colour changes through
blue, green and yellow (as does the colour of bruises on the human body), but because
of the hair and pigment of the horse's skin they are not easily detected. This extravasation of blood may extend through the tissues for a considerable distance, and when
the bleeding takes place in deeper muscles and under their sheaths the changes in colour
may take place at some distance from the site of injury.

Lymphorrhagia (Excess of free lymph)

Lymphatic vessels may be ruptured so that lymph escapes into the tissues, but the
pressure within the lymphatics is only slightly in excess of that in the surrounding tissues
so the escape can only be slight unless it finds its way to a neighbouring cavity. This
escape can easily be stopped by slight pressure; nevertheless, its presence after injury

cannot be neglected, for if it becomes stagnant it tends to act *as an adhesive between any neighbouring surfaces which lie close together.*

Hyperaemia (Excess of blood)

The demand by the tissues for oxygenated and nutritive-laden blood varies according to their activities, but if there is an excess of this blood beyond what is required the condition is abnormal. Injuries of all kinds produce an excess of blood. When damaged, the blood vessels allow blood to escape into the neighbouring tissues. If at the same time the muscles are injured, their pumping action is affected and the flow into the veins and lymphatics is reduced, and the part becomes congested.

Gravity also plays its part in arresting the flow into the veins and lymphatics, and when the blood and lymph becomes stagnant these vessels become dilated to such an extent that the valves of these vessels become ineffective; so the congestion is further increased. (See Fig. 14).

Long-continued congestion of these fluids can cause fibroid induration—callusing—which means that the part so affected is always liable to a further extravasation of blood and lymph from slight injury.

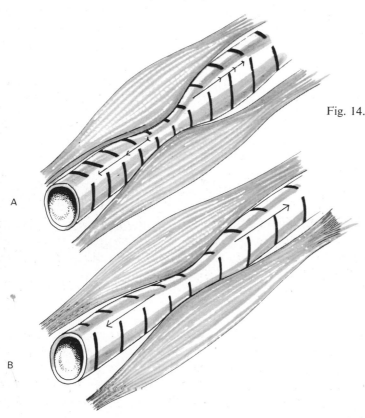

Fig. 14. A. **Lymph vessel,** B. **Vein.** (*Drawing, diagrammatic*). Showing the dilatation of these vessels to such an extent that the valve faces do not meet and so on compression of these vessels by the contracting surrounding muscles the fluid contents are not pushed in one direction only, as would be the case in a non-dilated vessel. This is a condition similar to varicose veins in the human

Local Anaemia (Local decrease of blood-supply)

A diminution of blood-supply is caused by anything which reduces or obstructs the bore of an artery. In the case of muscles and other tissues, contracting scars and inflammatory swellings taking place in dense strong tissues such as tendons, cause the same obstruction, decreasing the blood-supply. In the case of tendons this is very important on account of the already poor blood-supply.

The consequences of local anaemia, unless an alternative circulation (collateral circulation) is set up quickly, is that the surrounding areas become filled with non-circulating fluid. Coagulation then takes place and the tissue cells begin to die. (See Tendon Injuries, Page 74).

Atrophy of Muscle (Muscle wasting)

Under certain conditions, which will be described later (see Page 68) a muscle which is perfectly fit can become atrophied, by which is meant that it and its component parts become shrunk and emaciated. At a later stage its component parts become obliterated, going into a stage of fatty degeneration, making the muscle utterly useless.

The four main causes of muscle wastage are:—

1. Interference with the nerve supply.
2. Interference with the circulation.
3. Joint disease.
4. Disuse.

All degrees of muscle wasting take place if the motor nerve is damaged, whether partially or completely, for the motor nerve carries the stimulus to make the muscle contract. A muscle without efficient nerve-stimulus is like a motor without sufficient spark. As has been seen, if a muscle does not function properly, i.e. contract and relax, it wastes and degenerates.

In injuries to joints a great deal of attention is usually focused on the joint itself, but rarely do the muscles upon which the whole stability and function of the joint depend receive any attention at all. In acute or chronic inflammation of a joint, the muscles which habitually move that joint can no longer do so, and they lose their 'tone' and become wasted. Frequently, too, the muscles operating, and guarding, the joint may have been injured at the same time as the injury to the joint occurred. The joint and its muscles must have equal attention in such cases if full recovery is to take place.

Hypertrophy (Enlargement)

When a tissue shows enlargement beyond the normal it is said to be hypertrophied. In the case of muscle, if this consists of increased muscle tissue, it becomes capable of increased work. However, a muscle may increase in size and weight from certain causes owing to an increase in the amount of connective tissue at the expense of muscle fibres (muscle tissue). This is not a true hypertrophy because such a muscle loses the capacity for work. This condition is most usually seen in certain cases of paralysis in shoulders. Here, at first, the muscles will waste away completely and at a later stage the cavity, caused by the wasting, will fill up again; but this time not with muscular tissue, but with connective tissue which, from the point of view of work, is useless.

If a normal healthy muscle is made to contract repeatedly against moderate resistance (such as steady up-hill work) the muscle fibres will increase in size by the normal process of healthy development, until they reach a size requisite for the amount of work they are called upon to do. (So, after a horse is able to trot up-hill successfully the work is increased to cantering up-hill to build up yet more muscle tissue).

On the cessation of this extra work the muscle fibres tend to become fatty, the muscle becomes soft, flabby, less efficient and reduces in size. It is, therefore, less able to protect the joint over which it operates, from stress. To obtain an increase in size in a healthy muscle it is necessary for the muscle action to be repeatedly carried out against a definite resistance—such as steady up-hill work—and it is this extra work that is the main cause of the increased muscle tissue. Muscle activity alone, that is without resistance, does not succeed in increasing the size of a muscle beyond the normal, but such activity is beneficial as it keeps the muscle in a good state of 'tone'.

Rhythmic Muscular Contractions artificially produced by electro-stimulation can bring about an increase in muscle bulk beyond the normal (providing the correct technique is employed) but on ceasing to so stimulate the muscles they quickly lose the increased bulk and return to the size normal for the amount of work they are habitually doing. So there is little advantage in producing muscle development beyond what the horse requires for the job on hand.

General Effects of Injury

Injury acts as an irritant and produces inflammation. The effects of this can spread to a great distance from the seat of the original injury.

This inflammation is Nature's preliminary process towards repair, as it produces just what is required to effect that repair—an exudate or oozing of lymph to the injured parts.

As the exudate forces itself into the interstices of the tissues, the tissues become stretched so causing pain, and according to the degree of pain the animal rests the part, but only through the actual range of movement which is painful, provided he is allowed to move.

Repair

The object of the oozing lymph is to fill the space caused by the injury and join up the parted structures. The final result is an almost non-vascular, tough, *non-elastic fibrous scar* tissue. All would be well if this scar tissue formed only between the ends of the structures torn by the injury but, unless controlled, this new scar tissue forms wherever the exudate reaches, thus binding together structures (with non-elastic, tough fibrous tissue; in other words adhesions) which in normal conditions should work freely one upon the other. (See Fig. 15).

Inflammation

As has been seen, the inflammation comes in the first place from irritation of the tissue structures; produces local heat because of the increased blood supply, and possible chemical changes; produces swelling and pain, on account of the invasion of the exudate stretching the affected tissues—the actual pain being caused by the pressure on the nerve endings. There may be chemical changes also which affect the sensory nerves causing further pain.

During inflammation muscles function less well because they are restricted with exuded matter, and the nutrition of the muscle by fresh blood is reduced.

In chronic inflammation there is less heat, but the swelling is persistent and the formation of new adhesive tissue abundant.

Inflammation may be Nature's remedy in the natural state but, in the artificial state in which horses are kept, it requires guiding and controlling if the best recoveries are to be obtained.

The most important effects of prolonged inflammation may be summarized as follows:—

1. **Pressure Effects.** Excessive pressure on and stretching of tissues slows the local circulation, especially in the less elastic tissue such as tendons and the ligaments holding joints together.

2. **Hyperaemia Effects.** Cause dilation of the veins and lymphatics beyond their valve-efficiency standard. (See Fig. 14). It makes the muscular contraction and relaxation sluggish. Because of this pressure an excess of lymph exudate takes place.

3. **Hypertrophy Effects.** Some tissue elements are developed at the expense of others. In consequence they may shrink and have their capacity for work reduced.

4. **General Effects.** Muscles lose their essential qualities of tenacity, contractility and elasticity and begin to waste. With a muscle wasted and relaxed its tendons have to work at a disadvantage. Other joint structures—non-elastic ligaments and joint capsules —become stretched and lose their supporting qualities.

5. **Adhesions.** It has been emphasized that during the process of inflammation the exudate forces its way between the different structures, sometimes spreading some distance from the site of the injury. When this exudate becomes coagulated and changes into granulation tissue it sticks adjacent surfaces together. If the injured area is rested

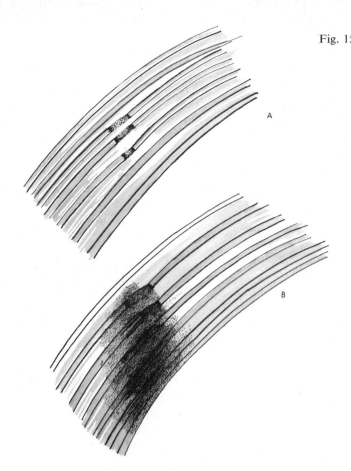

Fig. 15. **Torn tissues.** (*Drawing, diagrammatic*). No matter what tissue is involved—muscular, ligament or in fact any other—extravasation occurs at the site of the injury, to fill the gap and eventually form into scar tissue to join the torn structures together again

A. The ideal circumstances, where the exudate forms only between the injured structures

B. What actually happens. Not only does the exudate form between the ends of the torn tissues as in A, but it spreads between the surrounding structures, and if not controlled will form into adhesions—scar tissue —just where they are least desired. These adhesions not only limit movement but go on doing so to a greater and greater extent as time passes and as they contract

for too long a time these adhesions become stronger and hold the adjacent surfaces more and more firmly together. (See Fig. 15).

In the early stages these adherent surfaces are easily drawn apart. Later they become stronger, in fact so strong that movement is impossible. Adhesions may form in any part of the body, but especially so in the synovial linings of joints, tendon sheaths, in the connective tissue, so abundant in muscles, and in ligaments.

Joint adhesions may form inside or outside the joint, affecting its movement. Adhesions in muscles decrease their elasticity, and in other soft structures do harm because of their interference with the circulation.

Pain which precedes and accompanies the formation of adhesions aids and abets the evil process because it encourages the animal to keep the part still, while movement would prevent this sticking process.

From this it is obvious that to force an inflamed part to be kept an unduly long time at rest is only to assist this adhesive process. Properly controlled movements must be started before it is too late.

It will be shown that inflamed surfaces and parts can be kept on the move, and painlessly so, by electrical stimulation of the muscles. This not only prevents adhesions forming, but by moving the muscles not only is fresh blood-supply to the part increased but the venous and lymphatic return is stimulated, so preventing the inflammatory exudate from becoming stagnant.

Repair in Special Tissues

General principles of repair are essentially the same, but the more specialized the tissue the less easily is it repaired.

Connective tissue, such as that which pervades muscle, is capable of healing quicker and more completely than any other. *Elastic tissue*, such as that which makes up the vitally important suspensory ligaments, is capable of regenerating itself, but it is a slow job. However, these elastic tissues when damaged must not be over-rested, for so plentiful is the lymphatic supply in elastic tissue that when lymph is liberated it forms *non-elastic* adhesions—scar tissue. *Cartilage* is probably the slowest to reconstitute itself. *Repair of muscle* in slight cases presents little difficulty, but when scar tissue forms excessively, a more serious problem arises. (See Page 44).

CHAPTER IV

Strain

The words 'strain' and 'sprain' are usually used loosely to indicate injury other than fracture, but here the word 'strain' is used to denote injury to muscle alone and the word 'sprain' to define injury to the structures of a joint and to its muscles.

Muscles being elastic and contractile can put up with a great deal of pulling and stretching and no harm is done provided the muscle is strong enough (fit enough) to deal with the stress. However, when the degree of violence is so great that the muscle is injured, the damage may be confined to the muscle itself or may extend also to the ligaments of the joint which it helps to control.

A muscle may be injured by an effort that is successful in protecting a joint. As a result, although the joint structure has been saved, the efficiency of the joint becomes impaired because the injured muscle cannot now protect, or work, it properly. As a sequel to this, when a muscle is weak through injury the joint structures, i.e. the ligaments, etc., are vulnerable because they are no longer saved from stresses by the muscle. (See Fig. 16).

A common example of this is when the flexor muscles of a horse's forearm are injured or over-fatigued, as towards the end of a race; the fetlock joint is no longer properly supported and undue stress comes upon the suspensory and check ligaments, and this will continue so long as the flexor muscles remain inefficient. Again, the action of a group of undamaged muscles may be indirectly impaired as the result of strain to another group. (See Fig. 17).

When a muscle is strained it loses its:

1. Elasticity,	2. Contractility, and
3. Irritability,	4. Tonicity.

In a slight strain no actual damage is sustained by the muscle tissue but it loses its contractility and tone. It thus loses its alertness to contract to a sudden stress and so is unable fully to protect the joint which it works. Some of the muscle fibres may be slightly torn, the delicate connective tissue which pervades the muscle and forms the various sheaths may be injured. The subsequent bleeding and filling from the torn vessels which this connective tissue contains, no matter how small, causes discomfort

41

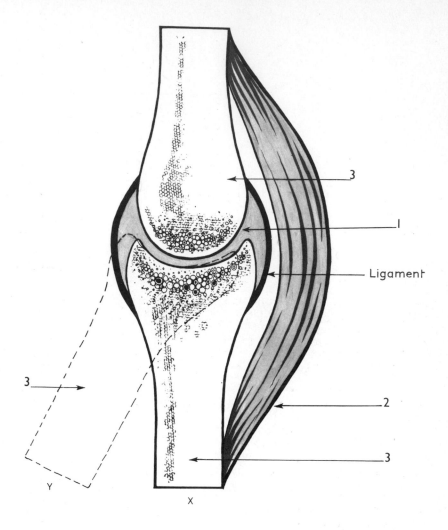

Fig. 16. **Longitudinal section of a joint.** (*Drawing, diagrammatic*). 1. Joint space, 2. Muscle which helps to operate the joint and guard the ligament from injury, 3. Bone. If the joint is moving from position 'X' to position 'Y'. Over movement in this direction is guarded by the muscle. Should the muscle fail to function correctly, stress will then fall upon the ligament. The muscle must either be overcome by the force which is moving the joint or be completely caught unawares and therefore off guard before the ligament can become injured. Therefore, if there is a weak muscle there is also a weak joint. Again, if there is a weak joint—i.e. an injured ligament—there is in all probability an injured muscle also. The joint cannot recover fully until the muscle is restored to full painless function. It is NOT possible to disassociate muscle injury from joint injury, or the reverse, no matter in what part of the body the injury takes place

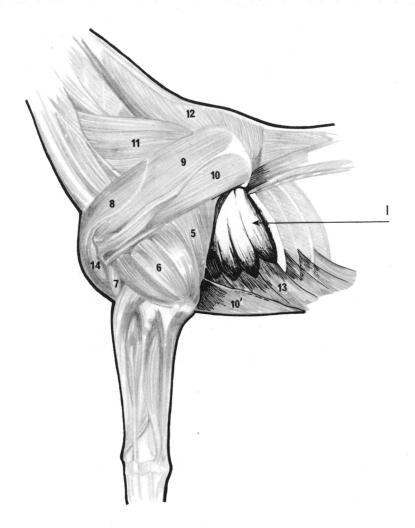

Fig. 17. **Deep layer of shoulder muscles, Lt.** (*Drawing, diagrammatic*). 1. Serratus thoracis, 5. Long head of triceps, 6. Lower head of triceps, 7. Brachialis, 8. Deep Anterior pectoral, 9. Supraspinatus, 10. Infraspinatus, 10¹. Posterior deep pectoral, 11. Serratus cervicis, 12. Rhomboids, 13. External abdominal oblique, 14. Biceps. Should muscle 'I'—serratus thoracis—be injured it will be unable to prevent the top of the shoulder blade rotating in an anti-clockwise direction when muscles 8 and 14—Anterior deep pectoral and biceps and other muscles on the front of the shoulder—contract to carry the leg forward. Reproduced from *An Atlas of Animal Anatomy for Artists* by W. Ellenberger, H. Baume & Dittrich. Copyright 1949, by courtesy of Dover Publications, Inc., New York 14, N.Y.

from the stretching of the affected part, and so causes lameness. If the strain is only slight the local tenderness and filling may escape notice altogether and, for example, if this slight injury occurs to a muscle on one side of the spine the only symptom the animal may show is a reluctance to turn to one side, the development of a tendency to jump to one side, the development of a preference to a right or left handed racecourse, to refuse when asked to jump or just show an unaccountable loss of 'form'. (See Fig. 6).

Some of these cases do get well by rest alone; or it would be more correct to say 'in spite of rest'. To rely on rest alone is to take a grave risk for if recovery does not soon take place the joint, or joints, become further crippled owing to muscle wasting, and the formation of adhesions becoming more numerous and stronger as time goes by. The joint becomes lax and the circulation to the surrounding tissues decreased.

The increasing seriousness of such a slight injury is mainly due to these after effects, and it is no uncommon history to have months of disability and pain as the result. Again, if the injury has escaped notice the animal may be classed as a 'rogue' or as having no courage.

This is well illustrated by a nine-year-old National Hunt racehorse which had shown considerable promise and which suddenly lost both form and jumping ability. He was presumably sound, but on account of his loss of form it had been decided he had lost his appetite for racing. As the author entered the box to see the animal he was informed by a responsible member of the stable staff that the animal was sound but quite 'gutless'. This despite the fact that this animal had earlier shown great willingness to both race and jump. There was no history of injury.

There was considerable rigidity of spine and finger pressure of the spine produced pain.

Diagnostic Rhythmic Muscular Contractions elicited painful muscular contractions in the muscles either side of the spine, especially on the right side.

Twelve treatments by Rhythmic Muscular Contractions restored free spinal movement and all muscles contracted free from pain.

At the time of writing this horse gallops and jumps very freely and his future career is anticipated with confidence. This horse has since raced three times winning two steeple-chases, one by a distance of twenty-five lengths, in very heavy going. Has since raced—over hurdles, and won.

Severe Strain of Muscle

In such cases muscle tissue is actually torn and also the connective tissue which ramifies throughout the whole muscle. The lymphatic vessels with which this tissue is so well supplied are torn, and coagulable lymph is poured into the surrounding tissues causing internal pressure and thus pain. There will be a considerable amount of blood freed from the torn blood-vessels.

The animal tries to obtain relief by holding the part still and in a position whereby the injured tissues have the least strain. As there is no movement, absorption of the escaped fluids is delayed and their stagnation follows. Adhesions form, further restricting movement. The animal continues to rest the part and so the adhesions become stronger. There is excessive muscle wasting and the case may, eventually, be considered incurable.

In the free state the animal would have to move the part, perhaps very slightly, if only to eat. This slight repeated movement might be sufficient to aid the absorption of the escaped fluids, discourage adhesion formation and decrease muscular wasting. At a later date a sudden movement in a moment of danger, or spurred on by hunger, he may pull free the adhesions. On the other hand he may become an easy prey to some predator.

In stable conditions early treatment is essential, as typified by the following case.

An internationally renowned show-jumper severely strained the muscles on the inner side of the right thigh (adductors). On the day following injury the part was so painful that he refused to move one step, and nothing would induce him to move. However, treatment by Rhythmic Muscular Contractions was started on the day following injury and on that evening, though lame, he could walk. He was treated for five consecutive days, by which time he was sound. A fortnight later he was show-jumping again—and winning at international shows—without trace of the injury. At the time of writing he has completed two further very successful seasons.

There can be little doubt that if this case had been treated by over-rest, and perhaps the application of heat in one form or another, all the dire consequences of neglected severe strain would have followed. (See Page 66).

However, not all late cases are hopeless. In most it is possible to pull free the adhesions by gently and progressively increasing the power of the contractions to the affected muscles. The freeing of adhesions in this manner does not cause as extensive an inflammation as rupture by more forceful methods, which must be resorted to in some extreme cases.

It has been reported that 'simple muscle strains usually recover with rest and some assistance from a liniment'. This, in some cases, may be so, but how is one to know how simple is the strain? What is thought to be a simple strain may with rest—and almost certainly with too much rest—turn into a chronic lameness. One may well be 'missing the boat' by not separating the adhesions soon enough. By leaving the condition too long the adhesions may become too strong ever to be pulled free.

A joint whose structure is quite normal may be weak and insecure for months because the muscles which operate it are wasted as the result of strain.

Joints treated by Rhythmic Muscular Contractions show, in the majority of cases, an increased stability in a few days, as the 'tone' and power of the muscles is restored.

The increase of power, taking place much sooner than any obvious increase in muscular tissue, gives the animal confidence to use the joint more freely.

CHAPTER V

Sprain

A 'sprain' as far as this book is concerned, is an injury to a joint whereby its structures in addition to its muscles have been injured as the result of a wrench or twist: the force of this may be so powerful or sudden that the protective action of the muscles concerned is unable to guard the joint. On the other hand, the muscles having lost their 'tone' or being still painful from a previous injury, are unable to do their job of protecting the joint efficiently. This latter can happen even if only a few fibres of a muscle, or a small portion of the elastic connective tissue which ramifies throughout the muscle forming the various sheaths, are injured and have made an incomplete recovery. (See Figs. 12, 15 and 16).

The structures which make up a typical joint are:—

1. Bones varying in number and shape according to their functions. These give support and act as levers.
2. Delicate cartilage, covering the ends of the bones, and acting as shock-absorbers.
3. Protective capsules of fibrous tissue, lined with secreting membrane, cushioning and oiling the working surfaces.
4. Ligaments of varying strength and size. These hold the bones together and limit their movement.
5. Arteries, veins, lymphatics and nerves. These are embedded in delicate connective tissue and fat.
6. Areolar tissue, forming cushions between the joint structures, and containing pads of fat.
7. Muscles of all shapes, sizes and strength enclosed in various sheaths of elastic connective tissue.
8. Synovial membrane whose secretion (joint oil) lessens friction.

If all these structures are considered individually and their relations to each other, it is obvious that when they are damaged the result may be as serious as a dislocation. In fact, a sprain is a momentary dislocation because, though the parts of the joint return to their normal positions when the stress of the wrench is over, for the moment they are truly dislocated. Otherwise there would be no stress on the ligaments, etc., and therefore no sprain.

On considering the mechanics of a joint, it is obvious that no two sprains are likely to be exactly similar. Some joints take the brunt of the stress on their ligaments, others, such as the shoulder, chiefly on their muscles.

When a joint has suffered a severe sprain, no matter how severe or what structures are damaged, the keynote of recovery is the rapid absorption of the effusion—or filling—which has taken place. The quicker this effusion can be cleared away the sooner will full movements of the joint be possible, and the joint return to its normal healthy state. Unfortunately, rest is usually the first procedure, and since rest does not help remove the effusion it does more harm than good. The longer rest is enforced so the possibility of full recovery is diminished.

The symptoms of an incomplete cure may be due to one or a number of causes, some of which may escape notice altogether. The muscles working the joint may be slightly or severely injured and have lost their 'tone'. The ligaments may become lax, except at that point where the structures were torn. The consequent bleeding and escape of lymph into the various parts, as has been seen, leads to adhesions in the capsule, tendons and muscles: not only in the actual structure of each, but between the other component parts of the joint, and this condition alone in the surrounding structures creates conditions somewhat similar to that of an injured muscle with adhesions forming between tissues, just where they are least desired and which as time passes become shorter and shorter further limiting movement. These may well be the cause of subsequent chronic lameness. (See Fig. 15 and case history on page 61). And in the case of injury to the suspensory ligaments the possible accompanying injury to the flexor muscles of the forearm may escape notice altogether, and without the efficient working of these muscles there can never be any hope of full recovery.

After rest, and most usually accompanying it, heat is applied, as it is thought that heat will bring more blood to the part and so aid the process of repair. But what is needed to aid the process of repair is an *increased circulation*. Heat will certainly, during its early application, bring more blood to the part, but it does little or nothing towards getting rid of the used blood and lymph *via* the veins and lymphatics. Heat, therefore, adds to the congestion and in so doing retards the process of repair.

By contracting and relaxing the muscles not only is a large amount of blood passed to the muscles and *all other neighbouring* structures, but it is also forced away by means of the muscular contractions pressing on the veins and lymphatics. This is one of the fundamental reasons why treatment of injured muscles and joints by Rhythmic Muscular Contractions gives such rapid and complete results.

It can be seen that quite a simple sprain to one part of a joint if inadequately treated by too much rest, and perhaps too much heat, can cause the part to become so clogged with blood and waste matter that the neighbouring components are affected. There is a saying 'Once a joint always a joint'. This is not surprising when in the past such inadequate treatment has been applied.

Just consider the natural consequences following the sprain. The blood-vessels dilate and at first the blood-supply to the part is increased. At the same time, the oozing from the torn capillaries, veins and lymphatic vessels, filling every available cavity. From this the synovial membranes become swollen, thickened and stretched, putting pressure on the nerve endings. There is an excess of joint oil mixed with blood in the joint cavity. The result is heat, pain and limitation of movement—in fact, what is known as inflammation.

The old belief that 'pain is Nature's cry for rest' when carried to excess has resulted in countless numbers of horses, and other animals, being 'written off' as useless, and often needlessly destroyed. Pain does cry for help, but for active help not passive help. No matter how severe the injury there is always a certain amount of movement which is free from pain, either in the joint or in the muscles which control it, and to ignore this painless range of movement is to court disaster.

During the period of reduced mobility it is essential to keep the muscles in action and the joint moving throughout the painless range of movement. This can be done painlessly by Rhythmic Muscular Contractions, when properly applied. The range of movement which is painless will increase daily and, in addition, the muscles upon which the joint depends for its security are kept in 'tone'. The effusion into, and into the structures around the joint is pumped away instead of being allowed to stagnate and form adhesions, and the horse returns to full work very much sooner than he would do by any other form of treatment at present in use.

Not only will the animal return to full work sooner, but the possibility of recurrence of the sprain will be almost non-existent as the muscles, upon which the security of the joint depends, are in good 'tone', are not wasted, and therefore able to carry out their function adequately. (See Page 68).

CHAPTER VI

Treatment by Rhythmic Muscular Contractions considered generally

The fundamental aim of treatment by Rhythmic Muscular Contractions is to restore movement to the muscles and to the joints.

By this means muscles and joint movements can be restored painlessly, even when the animal will not move the injured part of its own volition.

It has already been stressed that the physical and chemical changes which follow normal activity of muscles are essential to their well-being. In injured muscles and joints the artificially created muscular movements maintain this, and thus stagnation is avoided, circulation is restored, the waste products are removed by the stimulation of the venous and lymphatic flow. The swelling, heat and pain, caused by the effusion of blood and lymph, are removed quickly before they lead to adhesions. This, so long as the nerve path is intact, is achieved by Rhythmic Muscular Contractions. They, therefore, serve a triple purpose: get rid of the effusion, restore the circulation, and move the adhering surfaces.

At the will of the operator, the tendons, muscles and joint surfaces are moved, at first slightly, then gradually to a greater and greater range—and painlessly.

Here again, the effects of injury are recapitulated:—

1. All strained muscles lose their 'tone' and waste.

2. Strained and wasted muscles act incorrectly and in a limited manner with those of their group, so pressures on joint surfaces are unequal and, therefore, liable to undergo serious changes.

3. A joint with wasted muscles is at a mechanical disadvantage and liable to further injury from slight causes, as the weakened muscles are less able to protect it.

4. Wasted muscles mean deficient circulation, therefore joint surfaces are liable to structural changes.

5. The delicate connective tissue, well supplied with lymph, which fills up the interstices between the joint members is very vulnerable, and if injured creates pain,

causing the animal to rest the part. Consequently, adhesions form and further muscle wasting takes place.

6. Blood and lymph escaping into the injured part causes swelling, heat and pain and, unless this can be speedily absorbed, adhesions form. Over-rest only capitulates to this process, encouraging stagnation and adhesions.

Rhythmic Muscular Contractions if begun at once, and *painlessly*, should prevent the stagnation, anticipate the adhesive tendency and increase the circulation.

Even in severe cases of muscle and joint injury, necessitating the prevention of weight-bearing by the use of slings, the part should be made to work, painlessly, daily, to avoid the results of over-rest.

Horses sustaining slight muscular injuries which would perhaps recover with rest, or despite rest, need not suffer the set-back in their training schedule which accompanies rest, if treated at once.

Wherever there is a muscular injury there is a potential joint injury, if not already present.

One of the very great advantages with this method of treatment is that exercise can be combined with, and is an essential part of, the treatment. This means that many horses are in full work and, consequently, in something approaching fit condition for racing, hunting, polo, etc., on the completion of the treatment. In fact the horse should be brought up to full work as treatment progresses, and treatment continued until full work fails to reproduce symptoms of the injury.

COMPARISON WITH OTHER METHODS OF TREATMENT

In making comparison of treatment by Rhythmic Muscular Contractions and other forms, it is necessary to examine each and their individual effects.

It must always be borne in mind that the word 'circulation' means the function of the three systems as previously mentioned on page 25 and 28.

Rest. Though rest is sometimes essential in the early stages of an injury, complete or prolonged rest permits stagnation of the effusion and thus encourages the formation of adhesions. (See Page 49).

Cold. Contracts the blood-vessels and so, immediately after an injury, limits bleeding and effusion. Thus the pressure caused by the swelling is forestalled and the pain, to some extent, relieved. *It is of little use if applied after the effusion has taken place.* If applied at a later date it can only devitalize the part by reducing the circulation.

Heat. No matter how applied, i.e. hot poultices, hot fomentations, kaolin, diathermy, infra-red ray, radiant heat, ultra-short wave, inductothermy, microthermy and ultra-sonic (if the latter's action be that of heat) are all but different methods of applying heat. Some produce deep heat, others superficial heat, but none the less the effect is basically the same, i.e. dilates the blood-vessels and so brings more blood to the part but does little to stimulate the venous and lymphatic return. So, in fact, the circumstances are similar to the tremendous inflow traffic into a large city in the early mornings. So much traffic comes into the centre of the town, with so little going out, that in a very short space of time the centre of the town is so congested that there is hardly any circulation of traffic at all. Too much heat, no matter how it is applied, does NOT INCREASE CIR-CULATION OF THE BLOOD; as with the traffic, heat can cause such a congestion that it slows down the circulation, especially in the denser structures such as tendons.

It must be said, however, judicially applied heat is nearly always comforting; and it would be more comforting if the blood so brought to the part could be encouraged to return by the veins and lymphatics, but this cannot be achieved without muscular activity. (See Massage and Passive Movements).

Pressure. Especially if combined with cold, can limit the bleeding and effusion, and consequently reduce the circumstances which create pain; but to do this, it must be applied *before* the bleeding and effusion takes place. Once this has happened, pressure can only force the effusion into tissues not affected by the injury. Pressure, if applied after the swelling has taken place, and if accompanied by too much rest, will encourage the formation of adhesions not only at the site of the injury, but in the neighbouring tissues to which the pressure has forced the effusion. (See Fig. 15).

Massage and Passive Movements. Is the next best thing to treatment by Rhythmic Muscular Contractions, but it has to be carried out by a skilled operator. To fiddle about and tickle the skin is a waste of time—unfortunately, this kind of procedure often passes under the heading of Massage and Passive Movements. Skilful effluage alone achieves much more than banging, pinching and pushing, which, in fact, may do more harm than good.

Application of Various Lotions. If cold they can have little advantage over cold compresses. If their intention is to bring more blood to the part, the result is similar to heat treatment.

Blistering. Causes an increase of blood to the part. Its effect is the same as that of heat, only more drastic. The discomfort of the blister encourages the animal to rest the part and so increases the possibility of adhesions.

Hot and Cold. Alternately applied has some remedial value as it encourages circulation.

Charges. This procedure is similar in effect to that of plaster of Paris. It encourages stagnation and the formation of adhesions.

TREATMENT BY RHYTHMIC MUSCULAR CONTRACTIONS

In the case of a sprained joint, the joint itself is not directly treated, but controlled and rhythmic contractions and relaxations are applied to all the muscles which work on and over the joint. A start is made with the very slightest contractions which move all the muscles of the injured joint. By the end of ten to fifteen minutes all the movements have been gradually increased, and if the approach is made gradually enough it is very rare for the animal to resent the process; in fact, it probably works out that 75 per cent. like it, 24 per cent. tolerate it, and 1 per cent. dislike it.

Nothing is done to the joint to prevent bleeding or effusion, but as soon after the injury as possible, preferably the same day, Rhythmic Muscular Contractions are started. The effect on the joint is that there is an immediate increase in the CIRCULATION: STAGNATION of the effusions is PREVENTED by the muscular movements; absorption takes place actively; tendons and all parts of the joint inclined to stick to one another are kept on the move; the venous and lymphatic systems are stimulated. Muscle 'tone' is maintained and wasting prevented.

Obviously the sooner this treatment can be started the better, because the animal feeling the joint helpless and unreliable will not use it.

It might be thought that to use this treatment so soon after injury might increase the inflammation. Experience in the treatment of horses for some twenty years or more, and humans for over thirty-six years, shows that this is not the case. Not even in one single case has it been experienced.

Elastic Bandages. Before closing this chapter it must be stressed that, in the author's opinion, this form of bandaging is the most pernicious ever devised. It supports the muscles, and in consequence they waste to the same degree as they are supported. The pressure diminishes the circulation, and if the bandages are applied to the lower part of the legs during exercise and racing they reduce the circulation just at the very moment when it is most required.

It is a very different matter to pad and bandage the lower legs to protect them from bruising in horses required to jump.

CHAPTER VII

The Faradic Instrument

This consists chiefly of a means of producing a form of the faradic current of such a nature as to cause the least discomfort when applied to the skin and which is easily tolerated by the most highly-strung of thoroughbred horses, no matter what their stage of race-preparation may be.

The apparatus available at the time when the author decided to apply this treatment to horses, though suitable to humans as they could be persuaded in the interest of recovery to tolerate the discomfort, caused so much discomfort that horses in general would not accept it and an entirely new instrument was designed.

This has passed through many phases and the present instrument, called the 'SEVA', is ideally suited to the purpose.

After much experimental research it produces a current tolerated by 99 per cent. of the most highly-strung horses. It is absolutely safe in all stable conditions and is easy

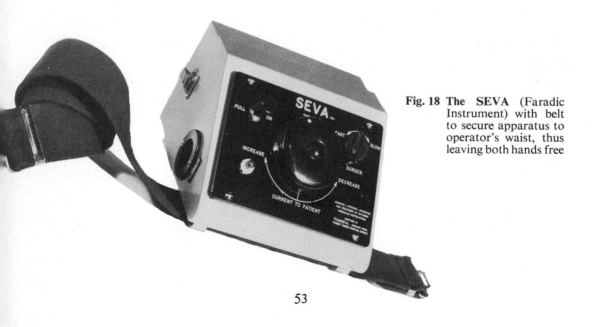

Fig. 18 The SEVA (Faradic Instrument) with belt to secure apparatus to operator's waist, thus leaving both hands free

to operate. The operator throughout the whole period of treatment has complete control over the strength of the contractions, their rapidity and the switching on and off of the current. There is no fear of an accidental and sudden increase of current to the animal, so frightening it, by movement of the horse or operator during treatment.

This instrument is now being produced by Messrs. Transeva, Jordans Farm, Forest Green, Dorking, Surrey, England, who at the outset discarded the idea of using the mains electricity supply as a source to operate the instrument.

In stable conditions both the horse and the operator are very well 'earthed'. Electrical instruments in the course of time, no matter how well made, might develop a fault, perhaps by rough handling, climatic conditions and ordinary wear and tear, and although the possibility of a short circuit allowing the full force of the mains supply to pass to the horse and operator is extremely remote, it nevertheless entailed an unacceptable risk.

The 'SEVA' is operated from dry batteries contained within the actual instrument, and the type of battery used is available throughout most countries. Thus the instrument is quite safe, no matter the circumstances or in what part of the world it is used. It is independent of all mains supply and the batteries as they become exhausted can be replaced quickly and easily.

This form of current goes on and off like the silent ringing of a modern telephone bell, but the duration, rapidity and strength is controlled by the operator. Whilst the current is 'on' it stimulates the muscle to contract, when it is 'off' it permits the muscle to relax and lengthen again to normal.

The sensation to a human being is as if the muscle is 'tweaked', then let go, then 'tweaked' again. With this particular instrument there is very little electrical sensation, if any at all. Some humans will describe it as a pleasant sensation and have been known to go to sleep during even strong treatment. One said of it, 'I now know what a clock feels like when it ticks.'

When the muscles have been contracted and relaxed for some time, the patient feels a sensation of decreasing tension in the injured area and, of course, this is just what is happening. Each contraction of the muscle pushes away some of the escaped blood and lymph which is causing the distension and pain.

According to the amount of current used, these contractions are strong or very gentle. The operator can make these contractions follow each other fast or slowly.

It is not, therefore, difficult to realise that with an instrument with such delicacy of control the muscular contractions can be applied with the greatest gentleness as in the case of very recent injury, or with vigour when it is necessary to push away stagnated effusions and to free structures bound together by old adhesions.

It must be repeated yet again, 'It is remarkable how highly-strung and 'corned-up' racehorses, of all ages, will show no resentment, except on very rare occasions, even on their first acquaintance with the sensation.'

54

The Faradic Instrument

It is not a form of massage. It is best described as a fully controlled form of artificial exercise which achieves in a fraction of the time the results which massage and passive movements, no matter how skilfully applied (and all other forms of treatment known at the present time) aim to achieve, but rarely do.

These are facts. *The apparatus does not heal*, but the effects of its use on the muscles create conditions wherein healing most easily takes place, i.e. increased CIRCULATION of the blood, and the active elimination of all those substances which, if left to stagnate, can sometimes cause permanent crippling.

CHAPTER VIII

Rhythmic Muscular Contractions used as a Means of Diagnosis

As mentioned earlier, the word 'strain' is used to denote injury to muscle alone, and the word 'sprain' is used to define the state of a joint in which any of its structures, besides the muscles, have been injured by a wrench or a twist.

As a joint in action is dependent on its muscles for its security, it follows that if any of these muscles are injured and lose their full efficiency, the joint is immediately at a disadvantage. And so long as the muscle, or muscles, remain in this state the joint is susceptible to recurring injury. (See Fig. 16).

It is, therefore, impossible to separate muscle injury from joint security, whether or not other structures of a joint have sustained injury. A joint cannot function efficiently so long as any of its structures, including the muscles, are in the slightest way suffering from the effects of injury.

In the more serious cases of sprain there are usually sufficient local signs in the affected joint to make diagnosis fairly easy, and one has then only to look to the muscles which control that particular joint to find which are strained. This is especially so when considering the joints of the four limbs below the level of the shoulder or hip. But should the lameness be due to muscle alone and no positive clue as yet is given by the joint, then diagnosis can be very difficult, especially if the offending muscle is above the level of the elbow or stifle.

However, this difficulty of diagnosis can be considerably reduced by using the method of Rhythmic Muscular Contractions to detect the injured muscle, or muscles; and once detected, cure can be effected by using the same Rhythmic Muscular Contractions in treatment as in diagnosis.

The current is applied to the horse in the same manner as for treatment, gradually increasing the current to contract each muscle individually throughout the whole suspected area. When an injured muscle is contracted, clear indications are shown by the horse flinching, raising the affected leg, or moving away, and a precise location of the injury can usually be defined. To confirm this, the corresponding muscle on the opposite side can be used as a control.

The experienced operator will sense at once when a muscle is responding to the stimulus in a manner different from the normal.

This, of course, does not exclude the essential 'nerve-block' to ascertain whether the foot is the main cause of the lameness.

In some cases of foot trouble the animal will use the limb in such a manner, to relieve painful pressure on the foot, as to produce muscular stress higher in the leg. It will be useless to treat this muscular condition if the main cause of the lameness is, after all, in the foot.

A 'nerve-block' is achieved by injecting a local anaesthetic (a 2 per cent. solution of procaine) in the vicinity of the nerves going to the foot, usually at a location just above the fetlock joint.

This temporarily kills all feeling in the foot. If the cause of the lameness is in the foot, the animal will go sound so long as the 'numbing' lasts. However, if he remains lame during the period of the 'nerve-block' the foot can be discounted as a cause of lameness.

In the case of so-called 'jarred shoulders' (where both shoulders are apparently affected and the horse goes with a short 'scratchy' or restricted action) it will be sufficient to 'nerve-block' one foot only. Should the cause of the defective action be in both feet, it will immediately show the horse as being lame in the leg not 'nerve-blocked'.

After 'nerve-blocking' there will most probably be a slight filling of the lower leg. This is of no consequence and will pass away, though it might cause a slight defect in the horse's action temporarily.

A 'nerve-block' to a hind foot is much more difficult and hazardous for the veterinary surgeon, than a fore foot and, of course, lameness in a hind leg due to foot trouble is much less frequent. So one is justified in treating a possible offending muscle, or joint, higher in the leg without previously 'nerve-blocking' the foot. But should there be no improvement after the second or third treatment then the foot must come under suspicion and a 'nerve-block' be carried out.

It must be emphasized that every muscle in the suspected area must be contracted individually; otherwise the vital one may be missed.

This possibility is well illustrated by a report from one of the most able lay users of this apparatus in Britain. 'A young horse was being broken-in—on long reins—when it reared and came over backwards and lamed itself badly in the near-quarter.'

It was treated immediately by Rhythmic Muscular Contractions on various parts of the quarter, inside and outside of the thigh, for two weeks without any improvement.

The operator was in despair of recovery but decided to give one more treatment. By sheer accident the mobile pad touched a small area between the spine and the stifle muscles. The horse resented this violently and immediately treatment was concentrated to this area. In one treatment the horse came out sound at the walk, and after three more treatments remained sound at all paces.

It sometimes happens after locating a possible faulty muscle that the first treatment might produce an increase in the degree of lameness. This is an excellent sign, meaning that the faulty area has indeed been located, but the first treatment has been sufficient only to drag upon the adhesions, making them more sore without freeing them. Further treatment will usually produce a cure.

CHAPTER IX

Cases suitable for treatment by Rhythmic Muscular Contractions

Broadly speaking, all cases of muscle and joint inflammation resulting from injury may be effectively treated by Rhythmic Muscular Contractions which, in addition to stimulating the process of repair, prevents the chief results of such inflammation, i.e., stiffness of joints, wasting of muscle, with the consequential insecurity of the joint upon which they operate, and the formation of adhesions in the joint, in the tissues around the joint, and in and between the muscles. Any or all of these may lead to a chronic lameness if not prevented by early treatment, or eliminated by the same, but more forceful, method of treatment at a later stage.

The very essence of the treatment is movement and, as the parts which have been injured may not be able to be moved voluntarily owing to pain, the method under description is particularly valuable because the necessary movements can be accurately controlled from zero to maximum according to the condition and what the animal can easily bear.

It is usual to classify suitable cases according to the structures injured and they are divided into the following groups with further notes on regional lameness.

GROUP 1. **MUSCLES**

A. Strain: (a) Slight strain.
    (b) Severe strain.
    (c) Strain resulting in adhesions in muscular tissues.
B. Haematoma in Muscle.
C. Contusion (Bruising).
D. Wasting of Muscle: from disuse generally.
E. Fibrositis (Muscular rheumatism).
F. Notes on foreleg lameness due to muscular strain.
G. Notes on hind leg lameness due to muscular strain.

GROUP 2. **TENDONS**

GROUP 3. **JOINTS**

A.   Sprain (Acute and chronic).
　　　　　　(a) Acute stage, immediately following injury.
　　　　　　(b) Chronic stage, resulting from adhesions.
B.   Sprain of suspensory ligaments.

GROUP 4. **STRAIN AND SPRAIN OF BACK**

GROUP 5. **DISLOCATIONS**

GROUP 6. **FRACTURES**

GROUP 7. **GENERAL DISEASES**

A.   Osteo-arthritis.
B.   Nerve injuries.

GROUP 1.   MUSCLES

As already stated, the word 'strain' is used to denote injury to muscle and the word 'sprain' to define injury to joint structures as well as to its muscles. Either may occur at the time of the injury. Should there be an injury to muscle alone it may be overlooked or, if discovered, dismissed as only a muscle strain or a 'pulled' muscle, owing chiefly to the difficulty previously experienced in making a precise diagnosis and of applying adequate treatment. There can now be no excuse for this as in the majority of cases, by using the diagnostic method of Rhythmic Muscular Contractions, it is possible not only to locate the particular group of muscles affected but the precise muscle most affected.

This is of importance when it is borne in mind that a joint cannot function efficiently when even one of its muscles is in a condition other than perfect.

It will be argued that some simple muscular strains frequently recover with no other treatment than a few days' rest. This might well be but, in the author's opinion, this is a grave risk to take, which is well illustrated by the following case:—

A National Hunt racehorse fell whilst racing, towards the end of a season; he was very lame, having injured the muscles of a forearm.

He was rested for a while and improved considerably; he was then 'turned out to grass' for a few weeks and eventually 'came in' presumably sound. He completed the following season's race-preparation of walking and trotting successfully, but as work progressed he was always lame after fast canters. A further few days' rest always restored him to walking and trotting sound.

A fortnight's treatment by Rhythmic Muscular Contractions brought no progress and he was destroyed. Post mortem examination showed that one of the injured muscles was almost entirely converted to fibrous tissue (adhesion tissue) which at so late a stage could never have been restored to normal contracting muscle. In addition, other muscles of the forearm were so strongly bound together by adhesions that it was impossible to separate them even with considerable force.

This condition was brought about by over-rest, and there is every possibility this horse would have been cured if only he had been treated by Rhythmic Muscular Contractions at once.

In contrast to this, another National Hunt racehorse fell badly whilst racing. He struck a fence and turned over vertically, hitting the ground with the left side of his head and his body rolled over to the right side, severely injuring all the soft structures on the left side of neck of shoulder. His immediate condition was so poor that destruction, where he had fallen, was considered. However, he was got home with great difficulty and X-rayed. There were no apparent fractures.

When seen the following day the horse was standing with the forelegs well apart; the

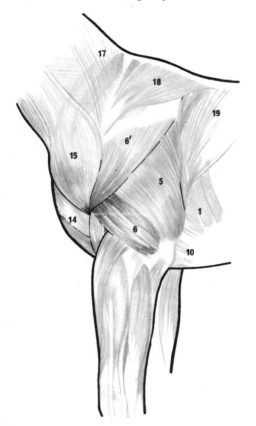

Fig. 19. **Superficial muscles of shoulder. Lt.** (*Drawing, diagrammatic*). 1. Serratus thoracis, 5. Long head of triceps, 6. Lower head of triceps, 6¹. Deltoid, 10. Posterior deep pectoral, 14. Anterior superficial pectoral, 15. Brachio-cephalicus, 17. Trapezius cervicalis, 18. Trapezius thoracalis, 19. Latissimus dorsi

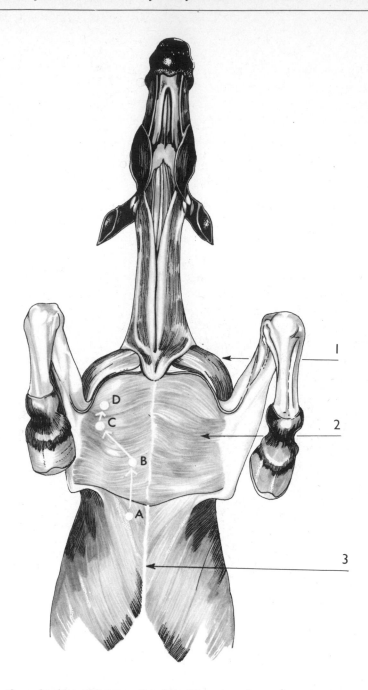

Fig. 20. **Muscles on the underside and between fore legs.** (*Drawing, diagrammatic*). 1. Brachiocephalicus, 2. Anterior and posterior superficial pectoral, 3. Posterior deep pectoral. The letters A, B, C and D relate to the text of page 105. (Ch. XI). Reproduced from *An Atlas of Animal Anatomy for Artists* by W. Ellenberger, H. Baume & Dittrich. Copyright 1949, by courtesy of Dover Publications, Inc., New York 14, N.Y.

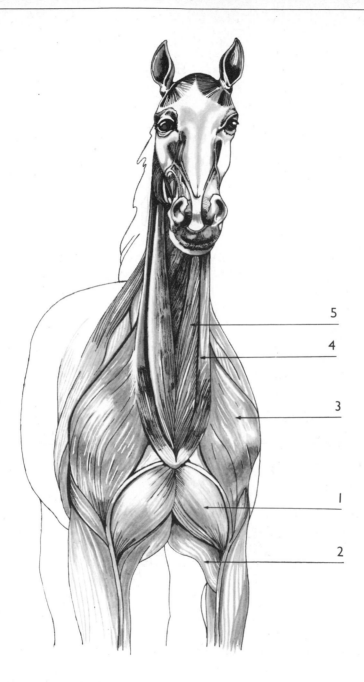

Fig. 21. **Muscles of fore-end of horse.** (*Drawing, diagrammatic*). 1. Anterior superficial pectoral, 2. Posterior superficial pectoral, 3. Brachiocephalicus, 4. Cutaneus coli, 5. Sterno-cephalicus. Reproduced from *An Atlas of Animal Anatomy for Artists* by W. Ellenberger, H. Baume & Dittrich. Copyright 1949, by courtesy of Dover Publications, Inc., New York 14, N.Y.

left knee was slightly bent, with the head slightly turned and twisted to the left and hanging so low that his chin was almost resting on the ground. Swelling extended from the withers and shoulder to the chin. The eyes were reduced to mere slits, and the ears partly engulfed by the swelling. The mouth was open with tongue protruding, and he was unable to move.

Treatment by Rhythmic Muscular Contractions was started some twenty hours after the actual injury, commencing with only the slightest contractions and gradually progressing to full strength contractions. As he became able to move he was encouraged to do more and more, progressing to normal exercise. Twelve treatments in all were given, and three weeks from the date of injury he galloped and jumped sound, showing no hesitation. A fortnight later he raced, and went on afterwards to win races without ill-effects from the accident.

On the other hand, horses have been successfully treated *after a period of twelve months' lameness* and have raced again with credit.

One such case was that of a 'classic contender' in a leading stable. His trainer considered him to be a very good horse indeed. However, he went lame in a hind leg during September of his two-year-old season. He recovered after a period of rest but was always lame after strong work, and this condition persisted throughout his three-year-old season. Nevertheless, he ran once but finished very lame.

He then came under treatment: diagnostic Rhythmic Muscular Contractions showed a strain of the hamstring muscles, and in eight treatments he was sound. Throughout the winter he was kept in reasonable work and as a four-year-old ran several times, winning twice and was placed on other occasions. All were very hard-run races, but he never showed further signs of the original, or any other, lameness.

As it turned out he was not as good a horse as it was thought. However, if he had been treated at the onset of the lameness, as a two-year-old, it is more than probable a cure would have been obtained in a matter of days, his training schedule not interfered with at all, and he could have taken his chances in the 'classics'.

There can be no greater mistake than *to see what a few days' rest will do*. In a few days it is remarkable how the escaped blood and lymph can stagnate, the oedema stretching the surrounding tissues, with the possibility of forming into crippling adhesions if the rest is continued and absorption does not take place.

A. Causes of Strain

If muscles, by their strength and correct timing, are able to overcome the force of a stress applied to them, they sustain no damage. But if the muscles are taken by surprise or are too slow in their response, or if the force applied to them is beyond their power of resistance, a strain of varying degree results. The injury is likely to be serious if the horse in endeavouring to recover slips again.

If the muscles are suffering from previous injury (possibly undetected), are unfit, or if they are fatigued at the time of the mishap, what might have been a trivial occurrence in a fit or untired muscle may result in serious disability.

This is particularly so in the case of the flexor muscles of the horse's forearm which when fatigued towards the end of a race, or caught unawares by the unevenness of hard ground, or suffering from undetected previous injury, are unable momentarily to take their full share of the animal's weight, then the stress falls upon other structures.

So, in addition to the muscular condition there is also a sprain most probably to the suspensory ligament, and so long as the muscular weakness remains uncorrected there is little hope of complete recovery. (See page 84 and Fig. 29).

All strains may be divided into three types:—

(a) *Slight Strain*

The affected muscle, or muscles, may merely be stretched; some of the muscle fibres may be slightly torn, and the connective tissue encasing the muscle fibres stretched or torn, with slight bleeding and escape of lymph, especially from the torn or stretched connective tissue. Even if the muscle is only stretched the principal effect is immediate loss of 'tone', with or without slight lameness. If lame, it quickly wears off with gentle exercise, but returns after a period of rest. On the other hand, there may be no lameness, and the condition shows itself only in a loss of 'form', a preference to a particular sided course, disinclination to jump, or jumping towards one side. The affected muscle, or muscles, is relatively lengthened and unable to contract fully so that it, and the joint upon which it operates, is placed mechanically at a disadvantage.

The onset may be sudden or gradual; if the latter, the condition may not be noticed at all and the loss of form attributed to the animal having lost his appetite for whatever his purpose may be, and so mistakenly classed as a 'rogue'.

Treatment of the affected muscle, or muscles, must be strictly within the animal's tolerance. Exercise must be maintained, but strong work omitted until the muscles are free from pain to the Rhythmic Muscular Contractions. A further two to three treatments can be given and then the animal tested at full work.

Defective action may be caused purely by a group of muscles having lost their 'tone' and therefore are not working in conjunction with others having, on certain movements, the same action.

An example of this was a six-year-old Arab show hack who, under close observation, was noticed just before taking the right hind leg forward, at the walk, to be rotating the leg inwards—rotating the hock outwards. On this being pointed out, the owner volunteered the information that the animal wore out the shoe on that foot more quickly than the others.

Investigation by the diagnostic method of Rhythmic Muscular Contractions showed the muscles on the inner side of the thigh—which in conjunction with those on the outer side carry the leg forward—were badly lacking in 'tone', and therefore were acting more slowly than those on the outer side, thus allowing the rotation of the leg. (See 'Contractility', Page 21).

Six treatments by Rhythmic Muscular Contractions restored normal action and he has since appeared successfully in the show ring. The wearing away of the shoes is now equal.

The condition was undoubtedly due to a minor injury of the affected muscles which, though recovering, had not regained their normal 'tone'. It is not known how long the condition had been present.

(b) *Severe Strain*

The onset is sudden. The muscle, or group of muscles, immediately loses its 'tone', and its power to contract is diminished according to the structural damage and the amount of bleeding and the escape of lymph into the surrounding tissues. This may spread through the tissues to a considerable distance.

The horse is very lame at once. Any sudden movement causes severe pain. A gap in the muscle may be detected and if the muscle sheath is ruptured some of the muscle may protrude causing a lump.

Treatment by Rhythmic Muscular Contractions offers the best probability of quick recovery and should begin at once, starting with the slightest degree of contraction to the *surrounding* muscles, and very gradually progressing on to those more affected. All treatment must be well within tolerance, progressing very gradually to full contractions to *all* affected muscles.

Severely lame animals might at first only be capable of walking a few steps, but this should be carried out several times a day and the distance increased at each period of exercise, or daily, in accordance with the condition. Treatment should continue daily till full work has been completed without any subsequent trace of lameness.

(c) *Strain Resulting in Adhesions*

This is due to imperfect recovery from severe or slight strain, especially if there has been much tearing of structures with bleeding and lymph stagnation in and around the site of injury; and more especially so if the part has been subjected to a period of over-rest immediately following the original injury.

The power to use adhering muscles (or the adhering fibres of an individual muscle) within limits is usually painless, but extreme movements, or movements suddenly carried out, produce momentary pain followed by a dull ache. Thus a horse which has sustained a strain of muscle (or a group of muscles) in which the absorption of the escaped fluids has not been complete may, after a period of rest, walk quite sound and even trot sound, but at some stage during progressively stronger work the adhesions will be pulled upon causing pain and consequent lameness. The ache and stiffness wears off to some extent according to the severity of the original injury, the period of over-rest, and the density of the consequent adhesions.

If the exercise has been strong enough to tear down some or all the old adhesions there may be a further escape of blood and lymph as in the original injury, and although this tearing-down of adhesions is a good thing if correctly treated at once, the condition will be worsened if the tearing-down of the adhesions is followed by a period of over-rest, which will allow the further extravasation to stagnate and so form more adhesions. There will be muscle wasting from disuse, which in some parts of the animal's frame may escape notice.

If adhesions are allowed to form after an injury and firmly establish themselves it is possible that subsequent treatment may only stretch them sufficiently to allow the horse free movement for so long as the treatment goes on: but the adhesions might again shorten, limiting movement, as soon as treatment stops, with a recurrence of the lameness.

This happened with an old hunter who had strained a shoulder-neck muscle and had been over-rested for a long time. He remained quite sound, and hunted sound, so long as treatment continued, but as soon as this was stopped the lameness returned.

Or as in the case of a two-year-old 'flat' racehorse who had been rested for a long time after sustaining a severe strain of left hind hamstring muscles. Treatment by Rhythmic Muscular Contractions produced a sound horse, but on returning to training always came-out in the mornings slightly stiff in that leg. This stiffness, however, wore off after a few minutes' exercise and in this condition he was able to win several useful races. He might have won more important races had treatment been started at once, and so produced a 100 per cent. cure.

B. Haematoma

A haematoma or tumour containing escaped blood varies in size and seriousness with its situation, and the amount and rate of bleeding from the torn vessels. It is usually caused by a blow. In the human, in its simplest form, it may occur after the pinching of a finger resulting in a 'blood-blister' where a rupturing of small capillaries has resulted. But in deeper tissues where larger blood-vessels are ruptured a greater escape of blood occurs and if this forms into a pocket of blood, creating a lump, it is known as a haematoma, or blood tumour. When severe it can necessitate an open operation to seal the torn vessels. On the other hand, if bleeding has ceased, Rhythmic Muscular Contractions to the surrounding muscles will usually bring about quick absorption.

C. Contusion or Bruising

Caused by a blow or the horse knocking himself. In minor conditions it may pass unnoticed and, if the horse is not stopped in his work, clear up completely. However, if there has been a severe rupturing of capillaries and lymph vessels, and if the subsequent extravasation is not rapidly absorbed and is allowed to stagnate in the area, adhesions may form restricting free movement of the structures involved in exactly the same way as a neglected strain or sprain.

If the flexor tendons of the forelegs are involved the condition may be serious, in fact just as serious as if the tendons had been strained.

An area sometimes involved is the vicinity of the 'pin-bone' (tuber coxae) from scrubbing on the floor should the horse be 'cast', insufficient bedding, or from striking this area on the door post when entering or leaving the stable. Here, again, all the consequences of an extravasation take place sometimes causing a hind leg lameness possibly of great obstinacy, especially if gravity has aided the extravasation to move downwards into the muscles which, at their upper end, are attached to this bone.

D. Muscle Wasting

Excluding certain diseases which need not concern us here, as far as sprain, strain and contusion are concerned, and providing the nerve supply remains intact, muscle wasting occurs only from disuse. Either the muscle, or muscles, is painful when contracted or when stretched, or by its contraction causes pain elsewhere. Relieve the cause of the pain, restore the muscle 'tone', and normal exercise will restore the muscle bulk and strength once more. Care, of course, must be taken during the muscle building exercise not to over stress the weakened muscles nor the joints upon which they work. (See Page 48).

Muscle wasting can be extensive and may extend upwards and as far forward as the muscles of the back if the animal has been resting a hind leg from any cause. Conversely, if the muscles of the back are injured and the horse has rested the hind leg on the affected side, muscle wasting and loss of 'tone' might extend to the whole leg on that side.

However, should the cause of the pain be strain, sprain or contusion and if this is treated early enough, the pain is relieved and normal action restored before muscle wasting can take place to any extent. Muscles wasted from disuse (either when directly injured or due to certain joint conditions), provided the cause of the pain is relieved, recover at a remarkable rate if treated by Rhythmic Muscular Contractions to restore their 'tone' and exercised to capacity. (See Page 48).

Nevertheless, muscle wasting in certain parts may be overlooked. Such as when it occurs in the forearm, back, between the front legs and on the inner side of the thigh.

E. Fibrositis (Muscular Rheumatism)

It is very doubtful if this condition is as common in horses as it is supposed to be. There is no doubt that many cases labelled 'rheumatism' are, in fact, the result of minor strain or sprain resulting from a diffused escape of blood and lymph into the surrounding tissues with the inevitable formation of minor adhesions. There will also be a loss of muscular 'tone'. These minor adhesions cause stiffness which becomes less with exercise, but should the exercise be insufficient to tear free the adhesions the stiffness will recur after a short period of rest.

Should the exercise be strong enough to drag free the adhesions and there is not a further escape of blood and lymph from this process, a cure might be claimed for the liniment which was rubbed on the part previously. This, of course, was purely incidental.

Should the exercise, however, in pulling free the adhesions cause a further escape of blood and lymph, and this is allowed to stagnate, there will be an increase in the severity of the symptoms.

Again, should the exercise be sufficient only to drag upon the adhesions without pulling them free, therefore making them more painful as the exercise continues, there will be an increasing lameness. This sometimes gives rise to 'Poor old fellow's rheumatism is bad today', or, 'The exercise yesterday didn't do his rheumatism any good.'

Treatment by Rhythmic Muscular Contractions and graduated exercise, up to full work, will usually clear up the condition quite rapidly.

F.   Notes on Foreleg Lameness Due to Muscular Lesion (Strain)

A horse was being cantered along the grass verge of a road when he put a foot in an unseen gully. The rider was thrown and the horse fell heavily on to its left shoulder. The rider was unhurt, but the horse got up very lame in its left foreleg. The owner was convinced that the lameness was due to an injury to the shoulder. The horse remained lame. Judging purely from the horse's action it certainly suggested that the shoulder could be at fault. However, before treatment was considered a 'nerve-block' was carried out. (See Page 57). The horse went sound immediately. This is a case within the author's experience and is told here to impress the importance of a 'nerve-block' to the foot no matter how obvious it may be that it is the shoulder muscles which are at fault. Incidentally, a subsequent X-ray of this horse's foot showed the navicular bone to be diseased.

However, should the 'nerve-block' fail to alter the animal's action, and there is no indication of injury between the foot and the knee, it is then, and only then, advisable to search the shoulder and forearm for muscular lesion.

The muscles of the whole area are individually contracted, going over the area several times, and if the lameness is due to a muscular lesion, muscles painful to contraction will be found. (See Page 56). This may be as far afield as the origin of latissimus dorsi, trapezius, serratus thoracis and cervicis, or brachiocephalicus. (See Figs. 17, 19, 21).

But the muscles most usually affected are triceps, deltoid, infra- and supra-spinatus, brachialis, anterior superficial pectoral or posterior deep pectoral. Strain of these two latter muscles, if present on both sides, gives rise to the condition generally known as 'jarred shoulders'. (See Fig. 20).

A good routine is to start investigation of a shoulder lameness from well back between the front legs on the affected side, forward and round under the point of the shoulder to the muscles on the outer side. If this proves negative, then to all the muscles attached to the shoulder blade. (See Fig. 17 and Fig. 19).

The muscles of the forearm are not frequently at fault, except in injuries to the flexor tendons, suspensory ligaments, knee and fetlock joints. In these latter injuries the muscles of the forearm are nearly always injured as well as the structures of the actual joint.

Unless these muscular lesions are corrected the joints will always remain at a dis-

69

advantage, with the possibility of recurring lameness until the muscular condition is cured.

In the case of recent injury, where the escaped blood and lymph are still fluid, the muscular contractions are kept strictly within the limit of pain. The horse should never show any resentment or more harm than good will be done; nevertheless, the contractions should be of such a magnitude as to be just short of causing pain.

In the case of old injury, where the escaped blood and lymph have become organized into adhesions, the muscular contractions have to be of such a nature as to pull free the adhesed structures.

Resistant strong adhesions (which should not occur if the injury is treated early enough) may sometimes have to be freed by strong exercise over a short distance. Increased lameness may follow from the subsequent effusion, but this can then be treated as a recent injury and the fluid absorption will be rapid and a cure obtained provided all adhesions have been freed. (See Page 91).

Once painless muscular contractions have been obtained and the animal is sound, normal progressive exercise will usually restore muscle bulk.

Throughout the period of treatment it is essential that the horse be kept in work as strongly as possible and just short of lameness. Very lame animals might at first walk only a few steps several times a day. But slightly lame ones should be given walking and trotting on good ground, and so on to faster paces, provided there is no deterioration in their condition. So, by the end of treatment, many will be fit for hunting, racing or polo, as the case may be.

As soon as the animal is sound at the walk, he can be ridden by a light-weight.

G. Notes on Hind Leg Lameness Due to Muscular Strain

In searching for the site of lesion in a hind leg lameness due to muscular strain the examination should cover the whole area from just behind the saddle, backwards to the top of the quarters, downwards to the muscles originating at the 'pin-bone' (tuber coxae). Then horizontally backwards to the tensor fascia lata, superficial gluteus, biceps, upwards slightly and further backwards to semitendinosus and so on to the semimembranosus.

Biceps femoris, semitendinosus and semimembranosus are the most commonly injured muscles of this area. (See Fig. 6 and 22).

If these muscles do not reveal any painful contraction then the muscles on the inner side of the thigh (adductors), high up into the groin should be investigated. This latter area is often the site of injury, and a severe strain here may make the animal stagger as he attempts to 'move over' in his box, in a manner similar to that of a slipping stifle. (See Fig. 23 and Fig. 24).

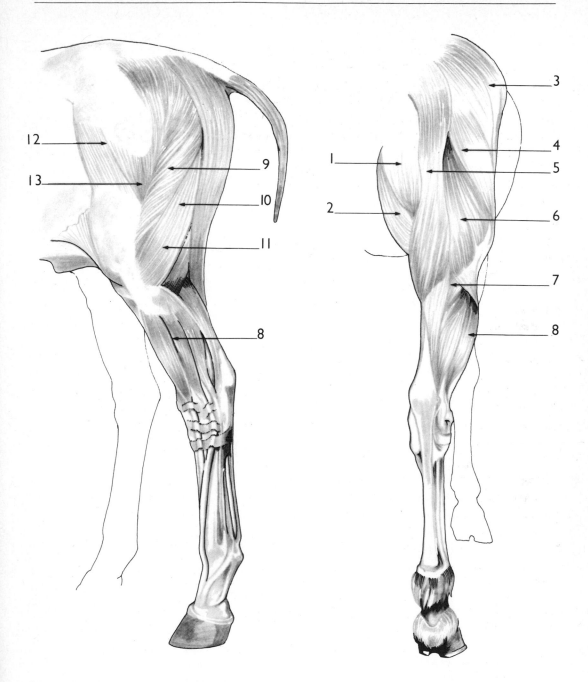

Fig. 22. **Principal muscles of hind leg.** (*Drawing, diagrammatic*). Outerside and rear aspects.
1. Semimembranosis, 2. Gracilis, 3. Gluteus maximus, 4 and 6. Biceps femoris,
5. Semitendinosis, 7. Gastrocnemius, outer head and just below this is soleus, 8.
Muscles which help to operate the hock and pastern joints, 9, 10 and 11. Biceps
femoris, 12. Tensor fascia lata, 13. Superficial glutius. Reproduced from *An Atlas
of Animal Antatomy for Artists* by W. Ellenberger, H. Baume & Dittrich. Copyright
1949, by courtesy of Dover Publications, Inc., New York 14, N.Y.

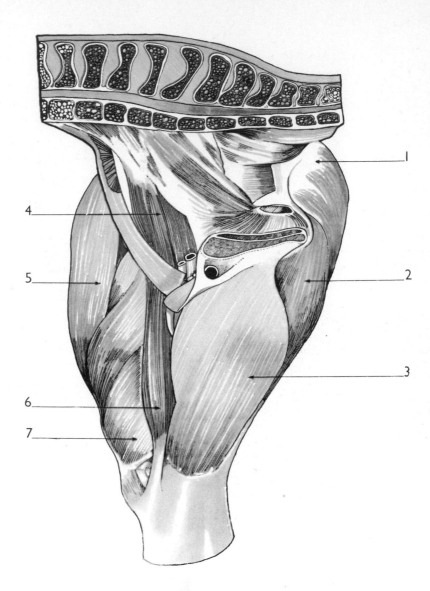

Fig. 23. **Principal muscles of the inner-side of thigh, superficial layer.** (*Drawing, diagrammatic*). 1. Semimembranosis, 3. Gracilis, 4. Iliacus, 5. Tensor fascia lata, 6. Sartorius, 7. Vastus internus, and just above this muscle Rectus femoris. Reproduced from Sisson & Grossman's *Anatomy of Animals* by courtesy of W. B. Saunders Company, Philadelphia, PA.

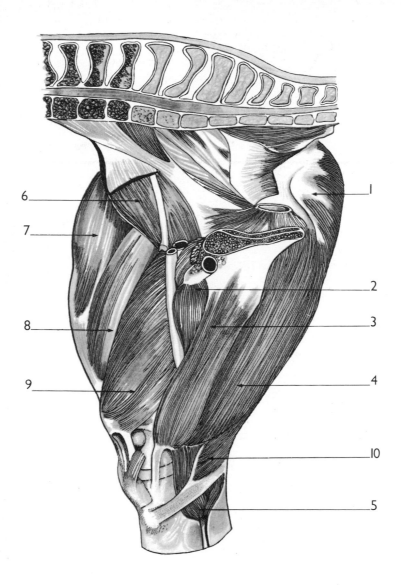

Fig. 24. **Principal muscles on the inner-side of the thigh, deeper layer.** (*Drawing, diagrammatic*).
1 and 4. Semimembranosis, 2. Pectineus, 3. Adductor femoris, 5. Gastrocnemius,
inner head, 6. Iliopsoas, 7. Tensor fascia lata, 8. Rectus femoris, 9. Internal vastus,
10. Semitendinosus. Reproduced from Sisson & Grossman's *Anatomy of Animals*
by courtesy of W. B. Saunders Company, Philadelphia, PA.

Group 2. **TENDONS**

Injuries to the deep and superficial flexor tendons of the forelegs, and to a lesser extent the less frequently injured flexor tendons of the hind legs are, perhaps, the most difficult of all horse injuries to deal with satisfactorily and within a reasonable space of time. The condition may be accompanied by injury to the muscles of the tendons, the enveloping synovial membrane and to the fibrous sheath.

As with the *suspensory ligament, the tendon structure is poorly supplied with blood vessels. It is, however, well endowed with lymphatic vessels and especially so in the deeper structure of the tendon.* It is important to keep in mind this poor blood-supply and the arrangement of the lymphatic vessels when considering the treatment of injuries to these tendons.

The actual tendon structure is not elastic, as is the suspensory ligament, and the elongation required when the horse's knee and foot are taken into full extension comes from the lengthening of the flexor muscles, of which the tendons are extensions. (See Figs. 25 and 26).

The tendon structure consists of numerous fibres running parallel to one another and when the tendon is at rest are somewhat wavy in appearance. This waviness disappears when the fibres are pulled upon and returns on the cessation of the stretching force. Therefore, though not elastic there is a slight 'give' in the tendons, and this may act as a form of 'shock-absorber'. It is this slight 'give' which may be the crucial factor in the treatment of these injuries.

At the time of the injury, and it is of little consequence whether the injury is caused by a blow (over-reaching) or a stretching force, lymph and blood-vessels situated deep within the tendon structure are ruptured and from these ruptured vessels their fluid contents (blood and lymph) escape: if this escape of blood and lymph could be limited strictly to between the torn fibres all would be well, *but it oozes between and around the surrounding tendon fibres and the blood- and lymph-vessels*, especially between the latter as they are more numerous, and this condition alone in the structures adjacent to the actual injury creates conditions somewhat similar to that of an injured muscle, with adhesions forming between tissues just where they are least desired. These may well be the cause of subsequent chronic lameness. (See Fig. 15). This escape of blood and lymph is proportionate to the degree of injury, and the synovial membrane and the tendon sheath may be involved.

If the injury is slight and occurs early during a period of exercise, the muscular activity of the upper leg (the alternate stretching and shortening of the lymphatics within the actual tendon, permitted by the wavy structure of the tendon and created at each stride taken by the horse) is sufficient to maintain a high degree of venous and lymphatic flow from the lower leg and so pump away the escaping fluid as quickly as it forms, and the horse returns to stables with completely clean legs.

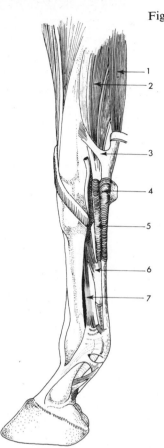

Fig. 25. **Principal muscles and structures on inner-side of horse's fore-leg. Rt.** (*Drawing, diagrammatic*). 1. Superficial flexor muscle—perforatus—2. Deep flexor muscle—perforans—3. Check ligament of superficial flexor muscle. 4. Superficial flexor tendon, 5. Deep flexor tendon, 6. Check ligament of deep flexor muscle, 7. Suspensory ligament. Reproduced from *Topographical Anatomy of the Limbs of the Horse* by O. Charnock Bradley and Tom Grahame, by courtesy of W. Green & Son, Ltd., Edinburgh

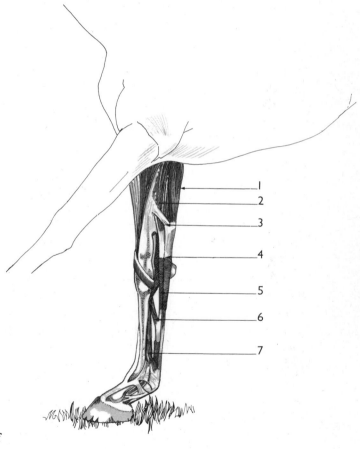

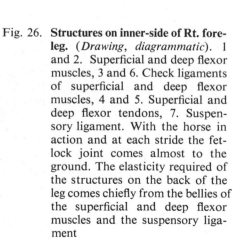

Fig. 26. **Structures on inner-side of Rt. fore-leg.** (*Drawing, diagrammatic*). 1 and 2. Superficial and deep flexor muscles, 3 and 6. Check ligaments of superficial and deep flexor muscles, 4 and 5. Superficial and deep flexor tendons, 7. Suspensory ligament. With the horse in action and at each stride the fetlock joint comes almost to the ground. The elasticity required of the structures on the back of the leg comes chiefly from the bellies of the superficial and deep flexor muscles and the suspensory ligament

75

However, during the period of rest following the exercise, throughout which the leg is, to a great extent, deprived of this muscular pumping action and of the alternate *pressures* and stretchings on and of the lymphatic vessels within the tendon, the lymph continues to escape and *collects in the vicinity of the site of the injury*—thus producing a localized swelling, heat and tenderness, but possibly no lameness even when the horse is trotted.

If this condition is ignored, in the case of horses used for fast work, and the horse continues to be galloped, favouring slightly the injured leg, it will most certainly be followed by a severe injury and both legs might be affected.

So it is known that to continue strong work will make the condition worse and therefore, in the past, the other extreme has been adopted as a form of treatment, i.e., rest, over-rest combined with applications of various lotions, various methods of applying heat, and various methods of applying cold, but all of them accompanied by rest.

There is a certain merit in applying cold and pressure, but *this must be applied before the swelling takes place*. It is of little use once the swelling has occurred. (See page 50).

If the injured leg is over-rested, with the tendon fibres unstretched (i.e. in their wavy appearance position), and there is little or no muscular action in the upper part of the leg or *those movements in the lower part of the leg which stimulate the lymphatic return*, then the escaping lymph will stagnate, as it is bound to do, and turn into adhesions binding together the tendon fibres (in their wavy position) and lymphatic vessels and, at the same time, perhaps, the synovial and fibrous sheaths. Indeed it can bind together all those surfaces between which it finds its way, which in the normal condition should move freely on one another at each stride of the horse.

In addition to this, if the injury is immediately followed by applications to the lower leg designed to stimulate the flow of BLOOD TO THE PART, and NO EFFORT IS MADE TO INCREASE THE VENOUS AND LYMPH FLOW FROM THE PART, there will be a further increase of escaping lymph to create more and denser adhesions with increased thickening of the tendon.

In due course the horse is gradually returned to work and as the work increases the adhesions are pulled upon. These being less extensible than their surrounding structures, further lymph-vessels are ruptured with a resulting further escape of lymph, and so a return of the original symptoms, perhaps with an extension of torn tendon fibres. In consequence, there will be a greater thickening of the tendon and its free movement within the tendon-sheath even more restricted.

Some little time ago it was found that operating on the tendon sheath, slitting it longitudinally to 'let-out the adhesive substance', offered the promise of improvement in results when compared to those treated by rest, blistering and 'firing'. This operation also reduced the constriction of the sheath around a thickened tendon, but the results from this operation were not as successful as had been hoped.

More recently this operation has been extended, as far as the superficial flexor tendon is concerned, not only to the slitting of the sheath but to the longitudinal opening of the actual tendon. Here a dead substance was found *deep* in the tendon structure, and just where the lymphatic vessels are most plentiful. Stagnated and necrosed lymph! (See Page 36.)

This is a considerable advance as far as old tendon injuries are concerned but would, perhaps, be unnecessary if the escaped lymph could be got rid of before it stagnated and so formed into this necrosed material.

Lymph flow from the lower leg is almost entirely dependent upon the activity of the muscles of the upper part; *the alternate pressure and relaxation of pressure on,* the alternate stretching and shortening of, the lymphatics deep within the tendon, created by each step of the horse. (See Fig. 11). As already pointed out, tendon tissue is very poorly supplied with blood-vessels. Nevertheless, repair of tendon injury depends upon a good CIRCULATION (see Page 25) and to bring about repair in the quickest time the circulation must be encouraged to the utmost. But this circulation is dependent to a great extent upon the muscular activity of the upper leg, and the movements so created in the lower part of the leg.

The passive application of heat to an injured area will certainly bring more blood TO THE PART, and can do so to such an extent that the subsequent congestion almost STOPS THE CIRCULATION. (See Page 50).

Therefore, it would seem if it is desired to *retard* repair and recovery of the horse the leg must be deprived of muscular activity by over-resting, and applying heat to the site of the injury. Tight bandaging will also aid in decreasing the circulation and by its pressure push the escaped lymph into surrounding structures not affected by the injury, so extending the area which can be affected by adhesions. (See Fig. 15).

It would seem, therefore, if a method of treatment is to be found to get these cases back into work within a reasonable time, or indeed at all, the solution may be found in striking a balance between:—

(a) Sufficient movement at the site of injury to prevent the wavy tendon fibres and lymphatic vessels, etc., becoming adherent to one another.

(b) Intensive muscular activity of the upper leg to stimulate a very good circulation; with special attention to the stimulation of the lymphatic flow from the deep structure of the tendon to prevent stagnation of the escaped lymph.

(c) Prevention of too much movement which would over-stress the injury and so increase the symptoms.

(d) It is also important to attend to the injury to the actual belly of the superficial and deep flexor muscles, which so often accompanies injuries to the tendons. Should this be neglected, and even if the tendon condition clears up, the muscles will be unable to take their allotted share of the stress when the horse is put back into work and an undue strain will fall upon the check and suspensory ligaments, with the possibility of subsequent sprain here as the result.

(e) If not searched for the muscular injury may not show itself till later when the horse reaches strong work, or even actual racing, when the extreme muscular effort drags upon the inter- and intra-muscular adhesions. The subsequent lameness is sometimes looked upon as a fresh injury when it may, in fact, be due to the neglected muscular injury which occurred at the time of the original injury to the tendons.

A sequel to this unresolved muscular condition is that, even if the tendon recovered, the horse in favouring the unresolved muscular condition of the injured leg takes most of the stress on the other and so injures this leg as well.

On the other hand, the leg can be 'fired' but recovery takes a very long time, the horse being out of action for the best part of twelve months, and this rules out the 'flat' racehorse in the majority of cases, and the muscular condition remains.

However, some very satisfactory results have been obtained by using Rhythmic Muscular Contractions, massage and graduated exercise: and, despite what has been previously said, the application of a hot poultice combined with the above, till the horse is sound at the walk. If there is no lameness at the walk the heat applications are dispensed with, BUT TREATMENT MUST START WITHIN TWENTY-FOUR HOURS OF THE INJURY—the same day being ideal.

The procedure is as follows:—

(i) If lame at the walk. Hot poultice and treatment by Rhythmic Muscular Contractions to all the muscles of the forearm, with special emphasis on the flexor muscles should these be injured. Treatment should be for sessions of half an hour, daily.

(ii) As soon as the horse is sound at the walk the hot poultice is dispensed with, and after treatment the horse is led out at the walk for an hour. This exercise, for half an hour, is repeated in the evening. Gradually extend the morning exercise to one and a half hours.

(iii) After each session of Rhythmic Muscular Contractions, and before evening exercise, five minutes massage is given. This consists of, and using a lubricant, firm upward stroking throughout the length of the tendons. (Effleurage).

(iv) As soon as the animal is sound at the trot he can be ridden by a light-weight and the morning exercise consist of walk and trot, whilst the evening exercise is restricted to being led at the walk. As much as possible of this exercise should be up-hill. This creates increased muscular effort of the leg and thereby increases the venous and lymphatic return.

(v) As soon as the animal is sound at the trot treatment is reduced to three times weekly.

At the end of about six weeks the horse should return to normal progressive work.

The best results so far obtained by the author, and incidentally the only ones which have come under treatment before stagnation of the escaped blood and lymph have taken place, are:—

A polo pony sustained a fairly severe tendon strain and of the fetlock joint. Treatment was started within two days of the injury and carried out on the above lines. Within six weeks the pony played fast polo on hard ground and continued to do so for the next three seasons without further sign of the injury.

Another case was that of a 'big-topped' high class four-year-old colt—a close fourth in the previous year's Derby—who sustained a strain of the 'off-fore' flexor tendons during the month of April. There was a tender soft swelling with heat at about the middle third of the tendons.

Treatment was completed and he returned to training within eight weeks. He went on to win at least three 'flat' races that same season. The leg remained absolutely 'fine' throughout his subsequent racing.

A similar case to the above was that of a six-year-old 'heavy-topped' entire 'flat' racehorse. He had strained the flexor tendons of the right foreleg early during the previous season. This leg was put in plaster for a while and he was rested for the remainder of that season. The following year, on being brought back into training, he strained the flexor tendons of the left foreleg on the 18th February. When seen two days later there was heat and a tender swelling some three inches in length in the mid-area of the tendons. The flexor muscles of the forearm were painful to Rhythmic Muscular Contractions. He was sound at the walk.

Treatment by Rhythmic Muscular Contractions and graduated exercise was started at once. Exercise was restricted to walking for one hour in the morning and evening (as described on Page 78) for seven days. He was then ridden by a light-weight, and morning exercise was extended to one and half hours, including trotting, with as much up-hill work as possible and this continued for six weeks.

At the end of this period the muscles had lost all tenderness and the tendons were absolutely 'fine' without any heat or tenderness, and he returned to normal training.

Within three months he had raced four times, winning once, and at the time of writing this horse remains sound.

A case of interest and one which serves to emphasize the importance of attending to the muscular strain which so often accompanies an injury to the tendons, was that of a five-year-old gelding 'flat' racehorse.

This animal as a three-year-old colt strained the flexor tendons of a foreleg. He was gelded and the tendons were 'fired' and he returned to training late in his four-year-old season.

He raced for the first time since the injury early in his five-year-old season, winning a very hard run race, but was lame afterwards due to an injury of the flexor muscles of the same leg. These muscles were swollen and tender to both touch and Rhythmic Muscular Contractions.

Six treatments to these muscles and graduated exercise restored complete soundness. He has since won on the 'flat'.

The author is of the opinion that the latter lameness was due to the rupturing of adhesions in the flexor muscles which formed following the original injury to the tendons.

GROUP 3. **JOINTS**

A. **Sprain** (Acute and chronic)
This heading includes all synonymous terms, such as:—
Arthritis (simple inflammation of joint due to injury).
Capsulitis.
Synovitis.
Windgalls.
Throughpins.
Capped hocks and elbows (Bursitis).
Jarred joints.
Sesamoiditis (without detached bone fragments).
Osselets.
Bog spavin, etc., etc.

(a)   *Acute sprain*, immediately following injury.

No matter which joint is affected; due to tearing of structures around the joint, blood and lymph escape into the tissues surrounding the joint and into the actual joint cavity immediately following injury.

If this free fluid is allowed to stagnate it forms into adhesions and, if not prevented, may cause permanent lameness; perhaps turning a simple arthritis (which is a simple inflammation of a joint and must not be confused with a rheumatic condition) into an osteo-arthritis.

The sooner treatment is started the better, no matter how severe the injury may be; in fact, the more severe the injury the more important it is to start treatment early.

Controlled contractions and relaxations of all the muscles which have an action on or over the joint, will cause the effusion to be absorbed and the wasting of the muscles will be prevented.

Even should the injury be so severe as to necessitate putting the horse in slings to relieve the joint of weight-bearing, early treatment is essential. It might only be possible to give the faintest contractions at the start but these should, and will, progress gradually to full strong contractions to all the muscles acting on or over the affected joint.

Muscles like all organs obtain a greater circulation of blood and lymph during activity than when at rest. The beneficial effects of electrically stimulating muscular activity of an injured joint has already been pointed out. (See Page 49).

As has been seen, the active circulatory changes hasten the absorption of the fluids and prevent stagnation, with all its consequences, to all or any of the joint structures and its muscles.

The results of this early treatment, when compared to the more usual method of rest, etc., can be described as nothing less than startling.

80

A polo pony who sustained a severe sprain of hock was seen two days after the injury. It had been rested with hot applications to the joint. There was considerable lameness; movement of the joint was limited by pain to about 90 per cent. There was acute tenderness on the inner side of the joint, and considerable fluid was present (bog spavin).

This case was treated by Rhythmic Muscular Contractions to all muscles with an action on and over this joint, together with graduated exercise. On the third day of treatment the pony was sound, there being no trace of heat, tenderness, fluid nor limitation of movement. The pony played fast polo within one week of the first treatment without further sign of this injury. Neither did he show any symptoms of this injury throughout the following three seasons of fast polo.

Another interesting case was that of a National Hunt racehorse who, whilst being 'broken' on long reins, reared right over and fell on his quarters, sustaining a sprain of hock. The following day he was lame with considerable swelling enveloping the whole joint, and he would not put that foot to the ground.

Rhythmic Muscular Contractions and graduated exercise produced a sound horse ten days later, and his 'breaking' proceeded without incident. He has since raced without further sign of this injury.

(b) *Chronic Stage of Sprain*

In this condition, prolonged effusion of blood and lymph into the ligaments and other tissues surrounding a joint and into the actual joint cavity has taken place, and there will be wasting of the muscles. Sometimes, in the case of a joint of a hind leg, the muscle wasting will extend as far afield as the muscles of the back. In the case of a foreleg, right up into the shoulder.

Such cases are of importance because owing to the weakness of the muscles which act upon the joint and the constant stretching of the ligaments (capsule) surrounding the joint from ever pressing fluid, the joint becomes loose and gradually and progressively less able to withstand the stresses to which it is subjected.

The flaccidity of the wasted muscles and the ligaments allows abnormal movement so that the fluid producing membranes of the joint (synovial membrane producing 'joint oil') are constantly irritated, with the result that further effusion of 'joint oil' is encouraged and more serious damage is liable to take place. When this occurs in the fore fetlock joints it is known in certain countries as 'osselets' or 'osslets' and in the early stages of the injury as 'green osselets'.

Absorption of fluid from the tissues surrounding the joint and from the joint cavity itself follows treatment, as soon as the muscular 'tone' is restored. The muscles increase in size and the joint becomes tightened which enables the horse to make further beneficial use of the limb.

It is remarkable how quickly long persistent fluid disappears when the muscles begin to recover their 'tone'.

In long-standing cases the adhesions both in the joint, and the ligaments surrounding the joint, and other soft tissues surrounding the joint, may have to be broken-down at some stage during treatment. But this should be necessary only in those cases which have been over-rested immediately following injury.

In some cases this might prove impossible and the condition is incurable. This is not the fault of the treatment by Rhythmic Muscular Contractions but the fault of it being applied too late.

Treatment is on the same lines as for an acute sprain, that is to all the muscles with an action on and over the affected joint, and to all the muscles which have wasted.

But whereas in the acute condition the muscular contractions are at all times painless, in the chronic stage the muscular contractions must be pushed to the maximum possible, but nevertheless strictly within the tolerance of the animal.

A horse, the winner of a classic race in his three-year-old season, early in his four-year-old season damaged both front fetlock joints ('green osselets'). He was rested and gradually brought back into work, but the condition recurred. It was feared that his racing career was finished and his immediate retirement to stud was being considered.

During eight days of treatment by Rhythmic Muscular Contractions his action improved daily. On the eighth day of treatment he won an important race at Royal Ascot, beating the previous year's Derby winner.

A case where it was thought the adhesions had become so strong that the condition might be irreversible was that of a brilliant heavy-weight hunter who had sprained the ligaments of a hind fetlock joint.

He was rested, but on return to work went lame. He was then blistered, but on return to work went lame. He was then 'pin-fired', but on return to work yet again went lame.

The joint was swollen, hot and tender, especially so when taken into a position of flexion. The condition was considered to be due to a sprain of the ligaments over the fore part of the joint, with subsequent dense adhesion formation due to over-rest and the consequential stagnation of the escaped lymph within the ligaments. (See Fig. 15).

Drastic methods were the only hope. The animal was given a short but very vigorous gallop, to break-down the adhesions, followed by long periods of walking and trotting. Each period of exercise the joint was sprayed with cold water for five minutes.

Within a fortnight he was sound and when last heard of had completed three seasons' hunting, in heavy country, without any return of symptoms.

B. **Sprain of Suspensory Ligaments** (See also Chapter IV, para. 4, page 41)

Injuries to the suspensory ligament are included under the heading of 'Joints' on account of their function, and structure, i.e. to prevent over-extension of the fetlock joint.

In the foreleg this ligament extends downwards from behind the knee, divides into two branches, and is attached just behind and to either side of the fetlock joint. Each

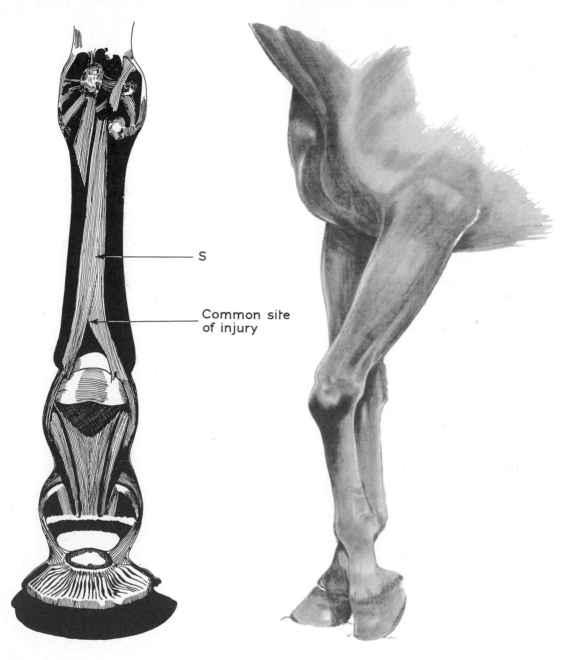

Fig. 27. 'S' Suspensory ligament of fore-leg, view from rear. (*Drawing, diagrammatic*)

Fig. 28. Horse resting Lt. fore-leg to relieve tension on structures in practically any part of the leg. (*Drawing, diagrammatic*)

branch then passes forwards and downwards, unites, and is attached to the front part of the pedal bone. In the hind leg the arrangement is similar, being attached above in the region of the hock joint. (See Figs. 25, 26, 27).

This ligament is of highly elastic structure and its function is to support the fetlock joint, with the aid of the check ligaments, when the flexor muscles of the forearm are in repose, and jointly (owing to its elasticity) with the flexor muscles and their tendons to flex the joint from the extended position. Again, when the horse is in action the extension stresses on the fetlock joint are shared between this ligament and the flexor muscles together with their tendons. (See Fig. 26).

Should (for any reason, such as fatigue, injury, or *being caught unawares*) the flexor muscles of the forearm fail to take their share of the extensor stresses, the full weight of the horse falls upon the suspensory ligament, stretching it to the full, and in so doing may tear some of the elastic fibres of which it is made; or it may split longitudinally at the point where it divides into two branches. (See Fig. 27).

The ligament, like the main ligament along the top-side of the neck, is made up of elastic-fibres, and similarly to tendon structure has an abundant supply of lymphatic vessels *but a poor blood-supply*.

At the time of injury not only are the elastic-fibres torn but the blood-vessels and lymphatics as well. If the escaping blood and lymph could be confined to the space between the torn structures all would be well (see Fig. 15) but it spreads and involves the surrounding structures. Thus the torn elastic-fibres, the torn blood- and lymphatic-vessels and non-injured surrounding elastic-fibres, blood- and lymphatic-vessels become enveloped in the escaped lymph.

If this escaped lymph, now surrounding the area of injury, is allowed to stagnate it . has a great capacity for forming into adhesions, which in this case form between the neighbouring ligament fibres and lymphatic vessels, as well as other structures. But, as already explained, these two structures have a high degree of elasticity; the adhesions, alas, have not this capacity.

Immediately following the injury, in order to avoid tension on the site of the injury, the horse will rest the part in a shortened position. (See Fig. 28).

If the flexor muscles are also injured at the same time, or just prior to, the injury to the ligament, there will be two sites of injury in which adhesions will form if the leg is over-rested.

No matter what treatment is applied to the ligament injury, if that of the muscles is neglected the chances of full recovery are considerably reduced. For when the horse is put back into work the flexor muscles are working at a disadvantage owing to their wasting from over-rest, and painful from the formation of adhesions; they, therefore, are unable to take their share of the extensor stresses, and the full strain again falls upon the suspensory ligament. (See Fig. 29).

Again, the adhesions of non-elastic scar tissue forming in the ligament are less ex-

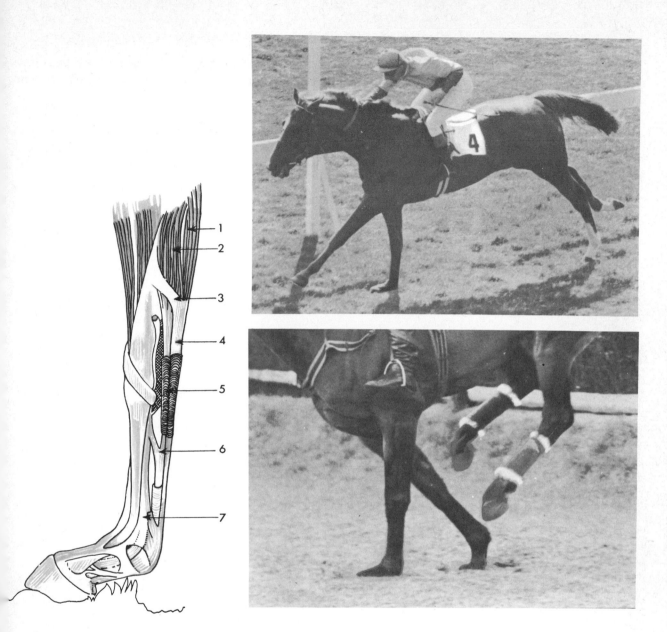

Fig. 29. **Inner side of Rt. fore-leg.** (*Drawing, diagrammatic and photographs*). 1 and 2. Flexor muscles. 4 and 5. Flexor tendons. 3 and 6. Check ligaments. 7. Suspensory ligament. At every stride when galloping, or landing over a jump, the fetlock joint comes almost to the ground. This stretching of structures on the back of the leg is accommodated chiefly by the muscles of the flexor tendons and the suspensory ligament. The strain is shared by these structures. Should, however, the muscles fail to function, extra stress falls upon the suspensory ligament and some of its fibres are torn. The tendons do not share this stretching as they are not extensible. Injury to the suspensory ligament is most likely to occur if the foot is UNEXPECTEDLY forced into over-extension by the horse treading—with his toe—on a hard mound, thus catching the flexor muscles unprepared for the extra stress owing to fatigue—as towards the end of a race—or weakness due to previous, not completely recovered, injury. Undue fatigue of the flexor muscles will also occur when these muscles are over-worked by having to pull the foot out of holding-ground at each stride. Eventually they are unable to take their share of the stress as the fetlock joint comes to the ground. And so a more severe stress is placed upon the suspensory ligament.

tensible than the structures to which they are adhered. So when the horse is put back into work this adhered area pulls upon the more fragile lymphatic-vessels tearing them, and there is an immediate further escape of lymph, and so the return of the original symptoms.

Treatment should aim at getting rid of the effusion and stepping-up the circulation, especially the flow of venous blood by means of the veins, and the lymph by means of the lymph-vessels.

Treatment should start WITHIN TWENTY-FOUR HOURS, the same day if possible, and the procedure is the same as for 'tendon injuries' but the hot poultice is omitted. (See Page 78).

Two cases, one a relatively fresh one, the other with a long history of recurring suspensory trouble, serve to illustrate the results to be expected from treatment by Rhythmic Muscular Contractions.

The first, a point-to-pointer, who had badly sprained this ligament in the off foreleg during preparation for the point-to-point season.

Treatment on the above lines was carried out·and he won a very hard-run point-to-point race within forty-seven days of the actual injury. He remained sound afterwards.

The second was a National Hunt racehorse who had been 'fired' for this injury three years previously and thereafter was always lame after steady work, and therefore could not be got really fit, and was never raced.

This horse was cured by treatment on the above lines. He subsequently raced, won once and was placed twice, without any return of symptoms.

In very old cases where adhesions are well established it might be necessary to break-down the adhesions by a short distance of fast work and then treat the resulting condition as a fresh injury.

The ideal, of course, is to start treatment the same day as the injury. The nearest the author has come to this was three days. Three treatments was sufficient to complete a cure. This horse subsequently raced many times on the 'flat' without further sign of this injury.

It is, perhaps, a little over-sanguine to expect a cure in a similar space of time in all such cases.

GROUP 4. STRAIN AND SPRAIN OF BACK

These are, perhaps, the most common of all horse injuries and undoubtedly the most frequently overlooked and neglected even if detected.

Arguing from what is known of the results of injury to other joints, for example the stifle, hock, knee and fetlock, it may be assumed that if an injury is of sufficient severity it will cause a similar condition in the joints of the spine, with the result that a simple synovitis (water on the joint) at the least must follow. The muscles controlling the movements see to it that little or no movement takes place in the affected joints and so adhesions are liable to form, not only in and around the joints and their ligaments but in the muscles also.

Cases suitable for treatment by Rhythmic Muscular Contractions

If the condition of a simple arthritis (inflammation of joint) is allowed to continue for too long a period it might then turn into an osteo-arthritis, and in the passage of time may become an actual fusion of the affected joint, or joints.

So what was a simple condition in the early stages may well become an incurable one if the part is over-rested for too long a period.

The method of pressure with the fingers over either side of the spine in the mid-area, immediately followed by a similar pressure just above the root of the tail, is of value in helping to determine the severity of the condition. But what appears to be free and unresented movement of the spine by this method is not decisive, as it does not indicate the lesser lesions which can cause so much trouble. (See Fig. 30).

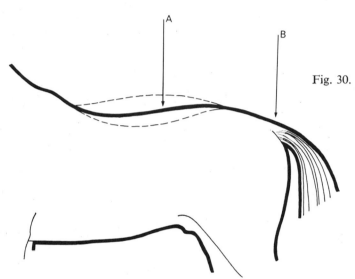

Fig. 30. In the normal condition there there should be free up and down movement of the back when finger pressures are applied to either side of the ridge of the spine at points A and B.(*Drawing, diagrammatic*). When pressure is applied at point A the spine will dip downwards, and when applied at B it will hump upwards. In this manner by using the left hand at point A, and the right hand at point B, it is possible —in the normal back—if the pressures are applied alternately to rock the horse's back up and down.

An example of this is well illustrated by the case of a seven-year-old 'chaser'. This horse fell during a steeplechase. He got up and seemed to be absolutely sound, but thereafter showed a loss of 'form' in as much as he frequently fell, and when he did complete the course showed no liking for the 'run-in' at the end of a race.

He was, nevertheless, apparently sound. Finger pressures over the spine showed free and unresented movement, and his condition was attributed to lack of confidence after the fall.

The muscles of his back were tested by the diagnostic method of Rhythmic Muscular Contractions and these showed a slight muscular lesion on the right side of the spine just behind the saddle.

This was treated by Rhythmic Muscular Contractions on six occasions, working up to strong contractions until all discomfort from this lesion was relieved. During this time he was kept in full work.

On his return home it was found he had regained his old 'form' and jumped very freely. He has since raced several times and has won four races of considerable merit.

A much worse case was that of a two-year-old filly who had injured her back, but there was no definite history of an accident; possibly 'cast' in her box. The condition had been present for some weeks and was not getting better.

She had difficulty in coming down the ramp from the travelling box. Her hind leg action was very restricted and 'tottery' and she would not turn except in large circles. Her back was rigid with no responsive movement, and she showed considerable resentment of finger pressure on any part of the spine behind the saddle.

When first applied considerable discomfort was elicited from Rhythmic Muscular Contractions to the muscles of the spine and top of quarter.

Twelve treatments by Rhythmic Muscular Contractions and graduated exercise restored free movement. She returned to training and has since raced, as a two-year-old, showing extremely free action, and has subsequently won.

A disappointing case was that of an eight-year-old 'chaser' who fell and hurt his back. He was rested for a long time and then turned out to grass for a season. When brought in he was still lame in a hind leg with a rigidity of back and muscle wasting extending from back to the lame hind leg.

A long period of treatment brought considerable improvement and he raced, but poorly. He was destroyed and the post mortem examination showed three bones of the spine fused together: the sad loss of what might have been a very valuable horse had he been suitably treated at an early stage.

'Cold backs', turning less freely to one side than the other, mouth one-sided, jumping sideways especially towards the end of a race, or preferring a particularly sided racecourse, and unaccountable loss of form, can frequently be attributed to neglected back strain or sprain, and if treated early enough a cure can be obtained in the vast majority of cases.   Sprain of the spinal joints and strain or contusion of the spinal muscles, either separately or all three combined, can be caused by a badly fitting saddle or the rider bumping heavily on to the saddle especially when riding with very short stirrup leathers. The subsequent action of the horse might be restricted hind leg action or loss of co-ordinated movement.

GROUP 5. DISLOCATIONS

Once a dislocation has been reduced it immediately becomes a severe form of sprain. In uncomplicated dislocations of all joints (with the exception of the joints of the spine, where in any case the animal will be destroyed at once) treatment of the muscles which have an action on and over the joint should start as soon as possible after the reduction of the dislocation.

An interesting case was that of a filly foal racehorse who dislocated a hind fetlock joint on the day of birth, and destruction was being considered. However, the dislocation was reduced and the joint put in plaster of Paris. This plaster lasted only a matter of days and this was substituted by bandaging.

Treatment by Rhythmic Muscular Contractions was started on the eighth day after injury, and was continued three times weekly for six weeks. After this the foal was sound, the limb was quite straight without any limitation of movement in the fetlock joint. As a yearling the horse attracted over £12,000 when sold.

This period of treatment could possibly have been reduced if treatment had started earlier.

Group 6. FRACTURES

Rhythmic Muscular Contractions can be of considerable help in all fracture cases but, of course, first of all every endeavour has to be made to ensure that the fragments are in a good, but not necessarily perfect, position for healing. Thereafter it is important to avoid stiffness in the joints above and below the site of fracture. In addition to this there is the possibility of adhesions between ligaments and muscles at the actual site of the fracture. If these become too firmly established the condition may be irreversible.

An important point is that Rhythmic Muscular Contractions so increase the local circulation that growth of callus is stimulated and union takes place earlier.

In cases of 'hip-down' (fracture of the tuber coxae) in the early stages, great caution should be taken not to allow the muscular contractions to further displace the detached fragment. However, after union or accommodation to the new position of the fragment has taken place, every endeavour should be made to get rid of the thickening in the soft tissues at the site of, and around, the injury. Other fractures of the pelvis should be treated with great respect and, at the risk of adhesions forming in soft tissue and between soft tissue and the site of fracture, left alone till bone union has taken place.

A happy ending to what might have been a hopeless case was that of a two-year-old filly who had fractured a bone at the back of the right knee (accessory carpal or pisiform bone). A long period of rest and 'pin-firing' had, perhaps, assisted union but no relief to the lameness. Four months after the 'firing' she was still lame, and bending of the knee joint was limited by about 50 per cent.

Twelve treatments by Rhythmic Muscular Contractions restored full movement and normal action. She returned to training and raced six times without further sign of this injury.

Detached fragments of the sesamoid bones at the back of the fetlock joints, if not a congenital condition (and if so are rarely accompanied by any inflammatory complications), should be treated as for a sprain of the fetlock joint provided the fragments are so detached as to be impossible of reunion with the parent bone, and are not free fragments which are likely to interfere with movement of the actual joint.

In a number of cases the fragments are deeply embedded in ligament and are unlikely to move further no matter what treatment is applied. So it is better to apply treatment for the ligament injury to prevent permanent thickening and the consequential limitation of movement.

GROUP 7. GENERAL DISEASES

A. Osteo-Arthritis

Resulting from injury. Is liable to occur from all injuries, and the older the horse the more likely it is to occur. It may be caused by a decreased circulation and stagnation of lymph resulting from injury; this affects the soft tissues, cartilage, and in due course bone. Bad function in varying degrees follows pain due to mechanical interference with joint movements by an excess of bone, adhesions and muscle wasting.

This type of osteo-arthritis benefits considerably from treatment by Rhythmic Muscular Contractions, but a complete cure is most unlikely. However, treatment of the injury in its initial stages by Rhythmic Muscular Contractions will reduce considerably the possibility of an osteo-arthritis supervening at a later stage. (See 'Back Injuries', Page 86).

B. Nerve Injuries

In general there are two types of paralysis: cases which are caused by nerve lesion above the level of the spinal cord (upper motor neuron), and the other type by a severance, bruising or the involvement of the particular nerve in the formation of callus around the site of bone fracture (lower motor neuron).

In the former, recovery is very doubtful and not within the scope of this treatment. The latter is of importance as in certain cases Rhythmic Muscular Contractions are of great use, if the motor nerve going to the affected muscles is intact. If, however, the nerve has been severed, or is deeply embedded in callus, recovery cannot take place until the severed ends of the nerve sheath are sewn together and the nerve has grown again throughout its full length or, in the case where the nerve is trapped in the callus surrounding a fracture, is released.

Should the paralysis be caused by a contusion (bruising) of the nerve then the greatly improved circulation brought about by Rhythmic Muscular Contractions can be of vital help, not only in relieving the pressure caused by the bruising itself but by artificially exercising the affected muscles until the nerve again takes up its full function.

In this manner the muscles do not waste to such an extent as would otherwise happen, and therefore remain in a state wherein they are able to take up their function again on the recovery of the nerve.

If the muscles are neglected throughout this period of paralysis they may degenerate into fibrous non-contractile tissue. So when the nerve recovery does take place there is no muscle tissue left for the nerve to function upon.

The two chief nerve conditions most likely to come under this treatment are paralysis of the supra-scapula and radial nerves, due to bruising. The affected muscles should be treated daily till the recovery of the nerve.

A point of importance is the maintenance of the mobility of the affected joints. Two cases of radial paralysis (dropped-elbow) were seen during one afternoon—both young horses. In both cases no effort had been made to maintain the mobility of the joints and, in consequence, the elbow, knee and fetlock joints were so stiff that even if the nerve had recovered the limb would have been useless owing to the stiffness of these joints. In both these cases, so stiff as to be irreversible.

Diseases of the Central Nervous System

Wobbler Syndrome

Shivering

Etc., etc.

Are unlikely to obtain any benefit from this treatment.

ANALGESICS

There is a strong argument in favour of the use of analgesics in the treatment of both acute and chronic painful conditions, but there is also a strong argument against their use for the following reasons:—

1. Acute stage. If analgesia completely relieves the pain, the animal might use the part so freely—and painlessly—that the extravasation continues and so the original condition becomes more extensive.

2. Chronic stage. If adhesions are pulled free during a period of freedom from pain, due to the analgesic, the horse might continue to use the part *too* freely during the period of an extravasation subsequent to the rupturing of adhesions: and so an extension of the original condition may ensue. In consequence the horse may be just as lame, or more so, on the wearing-off of the pain killing effects of the analgesic.

3. It is extremely difficult to treat an animal by Rhythmic Muscular Contractions if already under the effects of an analgesic. In the first place it is difficult, and sometimes impossible, to locate the precise site of injury or, on having found the site, of adjusting the degree of muscular contraction to that *just short* of creating pain.

4. The one advantage of an analgesic is in those chronic cases where Rhythmic Muscular Contractions have failed to pull free the adhesions and more vigorous methods have to be attempted. (See Page 70). However, the analgesic should be stopped as soon as the strong work has been completed, so that the subsequent effusion, due to the rupturing of the adhesions, can be treated as in the case of recent injury; that is, producing muscular contractions just short of pain. The effusion following these stronger methods is always much more severe than when it is possible to free the adhesions by Rhythmic Muscular Contractions.

CHAPTER X

Technique of treatment by Rhythmic Muscular Contractions

It cannot be overstressed that the following technique should be adhered to in every detail, to ensure that the horse, or any other animal, is caused the least possible amount of disturbance. Later, when the operator becomes expert, the details can be varied to suit the requirements of any particular case, or the requirements of the individual operator in the light of personal experience.

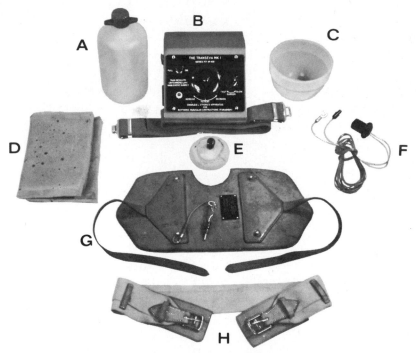

Fig. 31 A. Bottle of lubricant, B. The 'SEVA' faradic instrument complete with belt, C. Bowl, D. Indifferent electrode pad, E. Mobile electrode, F. Leads, G. Roller, H. Elastic girth

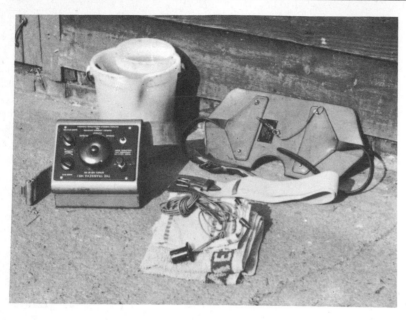

Fig. 32. The complete apparatus placed to one side of the entrance to the horse's box.

The complete apparatus consists of:—
1. The actual instrument, the 'Transeva'.
2. Special roller and elastic girth.
3. Pair of leads.
4. Mobile electrodes (2) Chamois leather covered circular pads.
5. Indifferent electrode pad—usually a large rectangular sponge-type pad.
6. A sponge.
7. Bottle containing lubricant paste for the mobile electrode.
8. Bowl.
(See Fig. 31).

In addition to the above, as supplied by the manufacturers, the following are required:

(a) a bucket.

(b) a towel.

(c) a snaffle bridle.

Place all the above to one side of the entrance to the horse's box. Bucket half-full of very warm water to which has been added a good handful of common salt.

In the following order place in the water, one of the mobile electrodes, the indifferent electrode pad and the sponge, and leave all three till quite soft. To aid the softening process they may be *very gently squeezed but do not bend till quite pliable.*

Half fill the bowl with the lubricant paste from the bottle and stand this on top of the contents of the bucket. In this manner the 'chill' is removed from the paste. (See Fig. 32).

93

With an assistant holding the horse by the reins of the snaffle bridle, remove the bowl to the side of the bucket. Take the well-wet sponge and thoroughly wet the saddle area of the horse's back, making sure the hair is well wetted down to the skin: this is very important when a horse has been 'roughed-off' to make sure that the dirt and grease of the horse's coat do not insulate the pad from the skin. Replace the sponge in the bucket.

Squeeze all surplus water from the indifferent pad, leaving it very well moist, and place over the wetted saddle area. Over this place the roller (metal plates downwards) and secure in place by means of the elastic girth.

The metal plates on the under surface of the roller must *NOT* be in direct contact with the horse. (See Fig. 33).

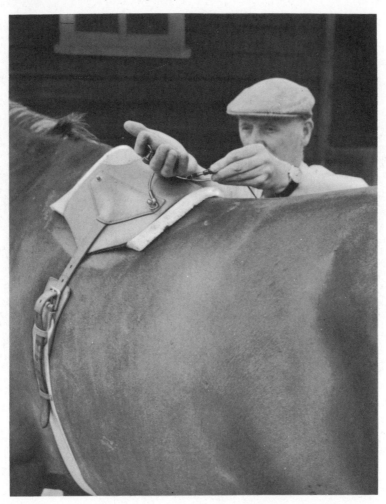

Fig. 33.
Make sure that the metal plates on the under surface of the roller are in contact only with the indifferent electrode pad. The metal plates must never make direct contact with the horse. Operator holding-down with the back of his Rt. hand the single pin connection of the roller, for inserting with the Lt. hand the single socket plug on one end of the leads

Technique of treatment by Rhythmic Muscular Contractions

From the bucket again take the sponge and well wet the hair and skin over the group of muscles or area to be treated. Return the sponge to the bucket.

Take the mobile electrode, squeezing from it all surplus water, and place it on top of the lubricant paste in the bowl.

Now take the bowl to the side of the horse, and on the mobile electrode take sufficient lubricant paste to cover the already wetted hair and skin of the treatment area. Rub the paste evenly over this area, adding more paste as necessary, until the mobile electrode runs smoothly over the hair. (See Fig. 34.) Replace the bowl, with the mobile electrode on top of the paste, at the side of the entrance to the horse's box.

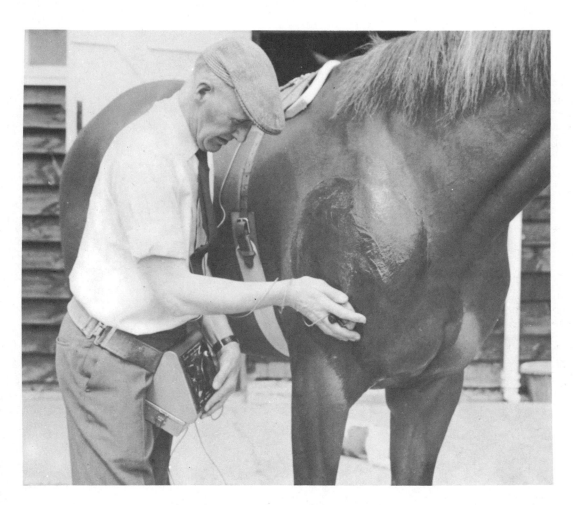

Fig. 34. Well lubricate the treatment area with the paste so that the mobile electrode runs freely over the surface of the animal's coat

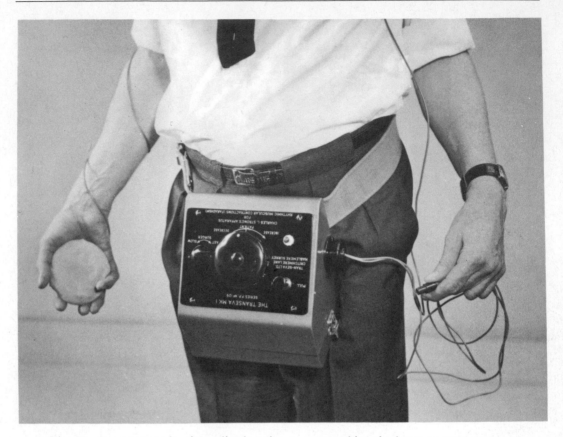

Fig. 35. Operator ready—immediately prior to approaching the horse to start treatment

Rinse the hands in the bucket and dry.

Whilst still at the entrance to the horse's box, strap the main instrument to the waist, buckle towards the right-hand side.

Unroll the leads and insert the multi-socket plug into the multi-pin socket on the left-hand end of the main instrument.

Ensure that the 'patient's out-put' control is at zero (that is, fully rotated in an anti-clockwise direction) and connect the spade-type terminal of the leads to the screw terminal of the mobile electrode. Secure firmly.

Holding the slack of the leads in the left hand and the remaining free end, with the single socket terminal, between the finger and thumb of this hand, take with the right hand a further supply of the lubricant paste on the mobile electrode and stand close to the horse. (See Fig. 35).

With the back of the right hand holding down the single pin terminal on the upper surface of the roller, with the left hand connect to this the single socket plug on the free

96

end of the leads, now held between the finger and thumb. (See Fig. 33).

With the right hand apply the mobile electrode to the treatment area.

Whilst moving the mobile electrode firmly over the skin with the right hand, with the now free left hand again ensure that the 'patient's out-put' control is at zero. (Fully rotated in an anti-clockwise direction).

Remove the right hand, holding the mobile electrode, from the horse and pull out the control marked 'pull on'.

Re-apply the right hand, holding the mobile electrode, to the horse and continue to move it over the treatment area.

Collect the slack of the leads over the left wrist. Some operators prefer to hold these lightly between the lips. (See Figs. 1 and 49).

Now place the left hand over the control panel in such a manner that the 'pull on' switch rests in the bend of the wrist with the fingers extended towards the slow-motion dial of the 'patient's out-put' control. (See Fig. 36).

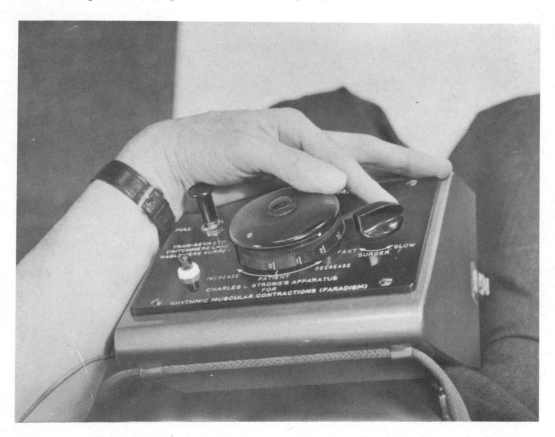

Fig. 36. Photograph taken from above operator. Correct position for operator's Lt. hand on control panel

Technique of treatment by Rhythmic Muscular Contractions

With the left hand now slowly turn the outer dial of the 'patient's out-put' control in a clockwise direction, and at the same time with the right hand continue to move the mobile electrode from place to place over the lubricated treatment area, until the faintest muscular contraction is felt by the hand holding the mobile electrode. Avoid any bony prominences and adjust the 'surge' control to give about 90/100 contractions per minute.

As the horse becomes accustomed to this degree of muscular contraction—usually a matter of one to two minutes—increase the current, but always slowly, to the amount desired and so continue to treat, varying the strength of the current to the amount required by each individual muscle.

As a general rule when treating recent injury, that is before the effusion has become organized, the muscular contractions should *NOT* cause the horse any discomfort.

In the case of old injuries, when it is desired to free adhesions, the muscular contractions should be full and strong, and especially so to the adhesed muscles. Nevertheless, the muscular contractions must be within the tolerance of the animal.

Move the mobile electrode from muscle to muscle, adjusting the current accordingly, and DO NOT GIVE MORE THAN SIX TO EIGHT CONSECUTIVE CONTRACTIONS TO ANY ONE MUSCLE. (See Page 24).

NEVER BE TEMPTED TO STRAP THE MOBILE ELECTRODE IN ONE PLACE, SO GIVING A LARGE NUMBER OF CONSECUTIVE CONTRACTIONS TO ONE MUSCLE OR, WHEN OVER A NERVE TRUNK, TO ONE WHOLE MUSCLE GROUP.

This is a bad technique as it presumes that all muscles are of the same size and strength and require the same amount of electricity to stimulate them to a given degree of contraction, which is not the case. This results in some muscles being over stimulated whilst others are being under stimulated. (See Page 24).

Each treatment should aim at giving at least about 3,500 muscular contractions, but treatment should stop at the first signs of muscular fatigue; due allowance being made for the loss of muscle 'tone'.

Though starting treatment at about 100 muscular contractions per minute these can be increased, but only as the operator becomes really experienced, to as many as 130 to the minute.

During treatment the mobile electrode must remain always in firm contact with the skin. Hold the mobile electrode well into the palm of the hand, with a turn of the lead round the wrist. (See Fig. 35).

In this manner the fingers and thumb are in contact with the horse's skin and the muscular contractions can be felt more easily. (See Fig. 34).

At the conclusion of treatment, reduce the current to the patient gradually by turning the 'patient's out-put' control to zero and then press fully home the 'pull-on' switch.

Disconnect the lead from the roller. Step away from the horse and return to the entrance to the box. Here disconnect the mobile electrode from the lead and replace on top of the lubricant paste in the bowl. Disconnect the leads from the multi-pin socket

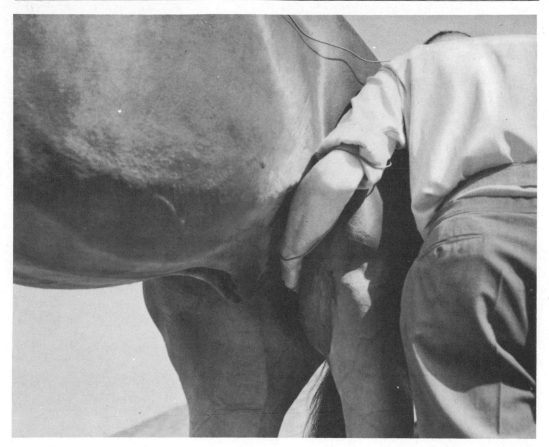

Fig. 37. The muscles on the inner side of the Lt. thigh are more easily treated if the operator reverses the use of his hands, i.e. the Lt. hand holding the mobile electrode and the Rt. hand on the control panel of the instrument

of the instrument. Roll up the leads and place in a safe place, near the bucket. Remove the instrument from the waist and place near the leads.

Return to the horse and remove the roller and indifferent electrode pad. Place the pad in the bucket and the roller near the instrument and leads.

From the bucket take the very wet sponge and wash from the horse *all* the remaining lubricant paste. Return sponge to the bucket.

Dry off the horse.

These instructions are given in almost pedantic detail, but it is the procedure of the author. In this manner the instrument and accessories are always together, and the operator does not move on to the next patient leaving some of the equipment behind. As experience is gained the operator can vary the procedure to suit his own requirements.

SOME NOTES ON TREATMENT

1.   Always allow about 10 seconds to lapse after switching on before increasing the current to the patient. This allows the instrument to reach full operational condition.

2.   To avoid accidental wastage of the batteries by leaving the instrument switched on, the internal circuit is broken on the removal of the leads plug from the multi-pin socket on the left-hand end of the instrument.

3.   Keep a firm and even contact with the mobile electrode during treatment or an unpleasant edge effect may be felt by the patient.

4.   If during treatment undesired muscular contractions occur under or behind the roller, remove the roller and replace further forward. Should the contractions continue, again remove the roller and thoroughly re-wet the saddle area. In the case of a horse which has been 'roughed-off', very well wet the saddle area to prevent the dirt and grease of the skin insulating the horse from the indifferent electrode pad and roller. This might also cause an uneven distribution of the current, hence the importance of well wetting the area.

5.   As the operator becomes expert the functions of the hands may be reversed according to which side of the horse is being treated. This is especially valuable when treating the adductor muscles of a hind leg. (See Fig. 37).

6.   The person holding the horse should always stand to the same side of the animal as the operator. So should the horse resent treatment its head, and not its hind-quarters, will be drawn towards the operator.

7.   Never treat a horse unattended, or securely tied up. Sometimes the quietest of horses will, for seemingly no reason, run-back.

8.   When treating a foreleg, the operator can place his head against the horse and so gently push the animal's weight on to the opposite leg. A cap should be worn when doing this to insulate the head from the horse, and so prevent the path of the current from passing by the head to the horse. This is a real hazard should the mobile electrode be accidentally removed from the horse during treatment. Not only will the operator receive a nasty electrical sensation through the head, but the horse may be frightened. This is of little consequence, but nevertheless unpleasant. (See Fig. 50).

9.   Take care to wash off all the lubricant paste after treatment. If any remains it will become hard when dry. This is of little consequence, but it is unsightly.

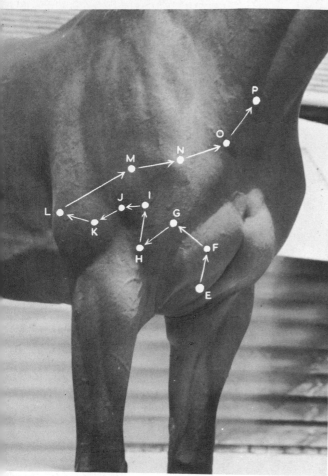

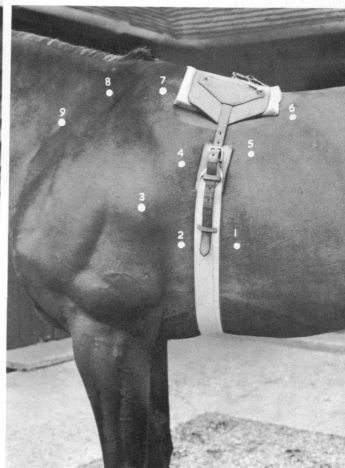

Fig. 38. Approximate location of motor points of muscles of Rt. shoulder. See text, page 105

Fig. 39. Approximate location of the motor points of: 1 and 2. Serratus thoracis, 3. Long head of triceps, 4, 5 and 6. Latissimus dorsi, 7 and 8. Spinalis dorsi and trapezius, 9. Serratus cervicis.

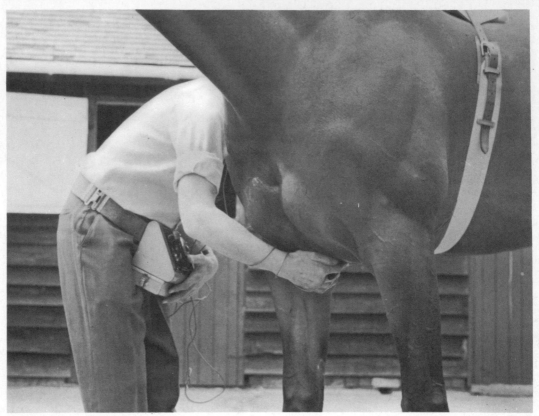

Fig. 40. Mobile electrode being applied to posterior superficial pectoral muscle of Rt. shoulder. Position 'D' of figure 20

10. The function of the small lamp on the control panel of the instrument is merely for testing the condition of the batteries, and is of no practical use from a treatment point of view, though it may flash as the current is increased to a certain degree.

11. It is an easy matter—and one requiring very little skill—to produce muscular contractions, even spectacular contractions which might impress the casual onlooker, but the art is to find the affected muscles and then to apply effective treatment to these muscles or to the muscles which control an injured joint.

It is of no use to produce muscular contractions, no matter how spectacular they may be, to one area when, in fact, the injury is in another.

The procedure consists, therefore, of two stages:—

(a) To find the affected muscles or muscle chiefly affected of a particular group. Having ascertained this one can then proceed to stage

(b) Actual treatment.

102

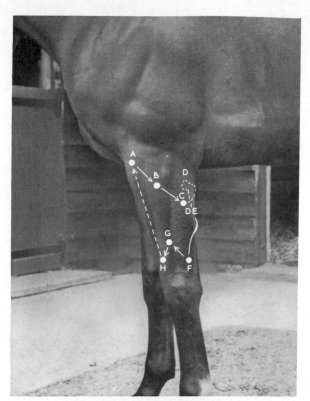

Fig. 41. Approximate location of motor points of the muscles on the outer side of the Lt. fore-arm

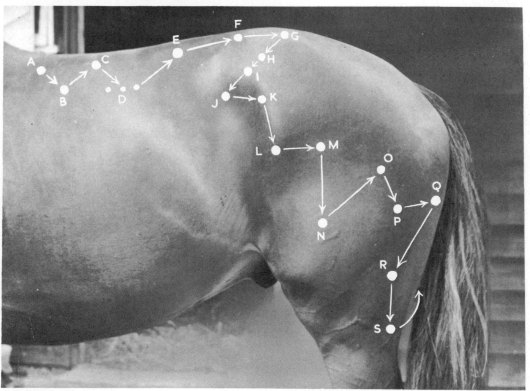

Fig. 42. Approximate location of motor points of the muscles on back and outer side of Lt. thigh

12. In the case of recent injury, where the effusion is still fluid, the most effective treatment is where the muscular contractions are as great as possible without producing pain. It is, therefore, essential to adjust the strength of the current to suit each individual muscle.

The most severely injured muscle requiring less current than the less severely injured muscles of that group.

13. More and more current will be required as treatment progresses.

14. In the case of old injury, where the effusion has formed into adhesions, the muscular contractions should be as great as possible to pull free the adhesions. Nevertheless, within the tolerance of the animal.

In view of the above it is impossible to give treatment of maximum benefit if analgesics are being administered at the same time. (See Page 91 'Analgesics').

CHAPTER XI

Notes on treatment to various regions

Motor Points are those positions on muscles where the muscle is most easily stimulated by the least amount of current.

These positions vary from animal to animal. So the positions indicated in Fig. 38, 39, 41, 42, 45, 47, are approximate, and are given only as a rough guide to the student operator.

In all Cases proceed as described in Chapter X. Before treatment can be attempted it is essential first of all to locate the precise muscle, or group of muscles, most involved and to ascertain this in the case of:—

Fore Limb Lameness—after the foot has been eliminated as the cause of the trouble— the whole chest and shoulder region is well wetted and liberally smeared with the lubricant paste to well back between the fore-legs. (See Fig. 34).

Now pass the mobile electrode well back between the fore-legs to a position as indicated by 'A' in Fig. 20, on the posterior deep pectoral muscle and start muscular contractions. Slide the electrode forward on to the superficial pectoral muscle at 'B', outward and forward to 'C'—anterior superficial pectoral muscle—and whilst at this position take the electrode slightly forward and outwards, on the same muscle, to position 'D'. (See also Fig. 40).

Then come on to the front part of the chest to position 'E' Fig. 38 and so on to 'P'. The whole time keep the mobile electrode in firm contact with the horse. At the same time watch the horse for indications of painful muscular contraction. As experience grows the operator will sense immediately the contraction of a painful muscle.

If this is not demonstrated at the first attempt, gradually increase the current and go over the whole area several times, producing greater and greater contractions.

If pain is demonstrated by the contraction of a particular muscle, this painful reaction can be confirmed by the contraction of the corresponding muscle on the opposite side.

In the shoulder area the muscles most frequently affected are the pectorals, especially

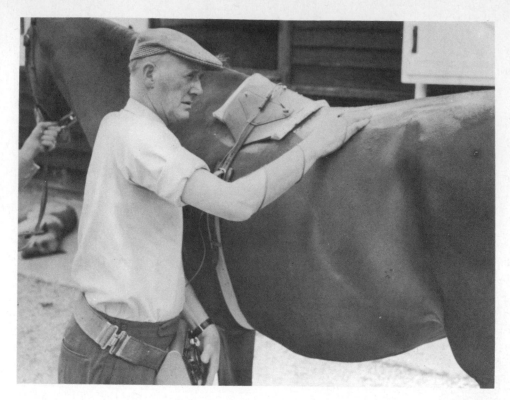

Fig. 43. Horse being treated for injury to back. Lt. side

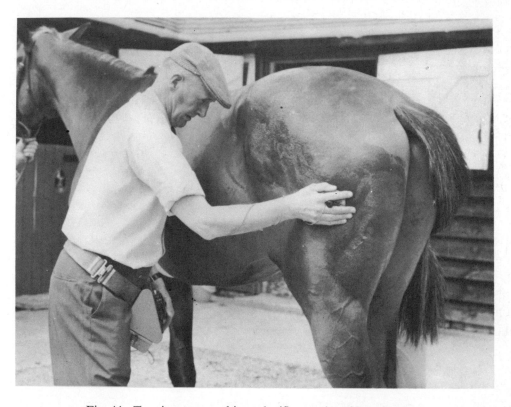

Fig. 44. Treating quarter, hip and stifle muscles of Lt. hind leg

at position 'D' (Fig. 20). Next in order of frequency are brachialis, deltoid and brachiocephalicus. The latter muscle at positions 'O' and 'P'. (Fig. 38).

Whilst at position 'M' slide the mobile electrode slightly upwards and in this position it is possible to stimulate both supra- and infra-spinatus. After these investigate serratus thoracis at '1' and '2', long head of triceps at '3', latissimus dorsi at '4', '5' and '6', spinalis dorsi and trapezius at '7' or '8', and serratus cervicis at '9'. (Fig. 39).

If these muscles do not indicate signs of injury proceed to the muscles of the forearm as shown by Fig. 41 and in turn contract all the muscles of the forearm individually.

When a muscle painful to contraction is found treatment is concentrated to the whole muscular group, with extra attention to the muscle, or muscles, most affected.

Hind Leg Lameness. Proceed as indicated by Fig. 42. Starting just behind the roller, progressing in the direction of the arrows. Contract in turn all the muscles of the back, quarter, outer side of, and back of thigh. (See Figs. 42, 43, 44, 45, 46). If these prove negative proceed to the muscles of the second thigh. (See Fig. 47).

In a one-sided hind leg lameness a muscle of the back may be the sole cause, but those most usually affected are biceps-femoris, semitendinosis, semimembranosis. If this last muscle is painful to contraction then the adductors of the thigh are usually involved also. Especially sartorius, gracilis and adductor-femoris. (See Figs. 22, 23, 24, 37, 48, 49).

Stimulation of the adductors of the thigh may be obtained by pressing the mobile electrode high into the groin and gradually sliding it from far back to well forward in an almost horizontal line. What seems to be ilio-psoas is sometimes affected. (See Figs. 48, 49).

Gastrocnemius and soleus must not be excluded from an investigation of a hind leg lameness.

Injuries to the Back. All muscles of the back, both sides, are searched as indicated by 'A' to 'H' in Figs. 42, 43. During this process it is best to contract the corresponding muscles on either side of the spine alternately. By this method it is very easy to compare the horse's reaction to each contraction and thereby gain a valuable and easy control.

When investigating, or treating, a back the operator stands on one side of the horse and reaches over the spine to the muscles of the opposite side.

JOINTS

Back. The various joints of the spine can be injured, like all other joints, with or without muscular involvement. However, no matter which is the case all the muscles of the back are treated from just behind the roller to the top of the quarters. Should there be any muscular involvement then extra attention is applied to those affected. (See Figs. 42, 43).

Notes on treatment to various regions

Shoulder. Treatment is applied to all the muscles which act on and over this joint. (See Figs. 20, 34, 38, 39, 40).

Elbow Joint. Treatment is carried out as for all other joints, i.e. Treatment is applied to all muscles of the region.

Knee and All Joints below this Level. Treatment is applied to all the muscles of the fore-arm, with special attention to those most affected.

The mobile electrode is never applied below the level of the knee, as there are no muscles below this level. (See Figs. 41, 50, 51).

Hip Joint. All the muscles with an action on or over this joint are treated with special attention to those most affected. Starting well back along the spine from 'E' (Fig. 42), to all the muscles of the thigh, outer, inner and back. (See Figs. 37, 42, 44, 45, 46, 47, 48, 49).

Fig. 45. Approximate location of motor points of hamstring muscles. Lt. thigh

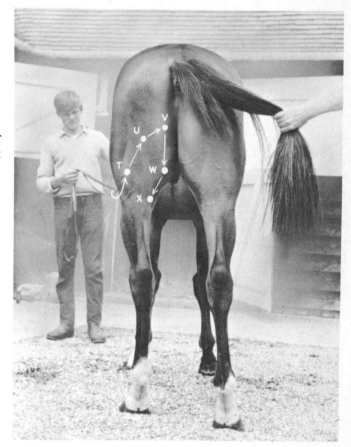

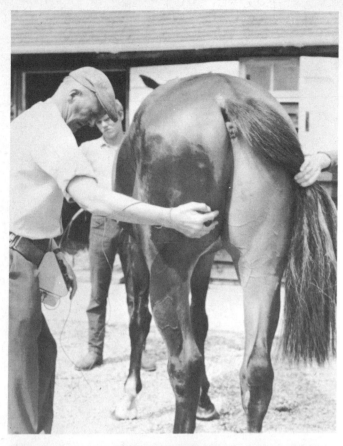

Fig. 46. Treating hamstring muscles of Lt. hind leg

Fig. 47. Approximate location of motor points of muscles of second thigh

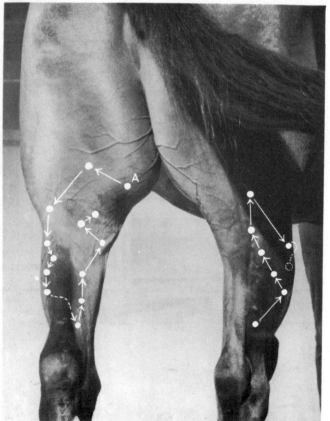

Stifle Joint. The procedure is the same as for a hip injury and always include biceps-femoris. (See Figs. 42, 44, 45, 46).

Hock and All Joints below this Level. All muscles of the second thigh together with the hamstring muscles, i.e. biceps-femoris, semitendinosis, semimembranosis and hindmost muscles of the inner side of the thigh (Adductors). (See Figs. 44, 45, 46, 47).

The mobile electrode is never taken below the level of the hock, even when the fetlock, pastern and coffin joints are being treated.

Flexor Tendons and Suspensory Ligaments of the Foreleg. (See Fig. 41).

All the muscles of the forearm are treated with special attention to the flexor muscles. Take the mobile electrode high up on the under side of the forearm close to the elbow and on to the chest in this region—posterior deep pectoral—in order to gain the greatest possible stimulation of the lymph flow.

Whilst treating these muscles the operator should with his covered head push the horse's weight towards the opposite side. The animal will then allow the leg being treated to hang relaxed with both knee and fetlock joints semi-bent, with the toe only resting on the ground. In this manner the most effective treatment can be given. (See Figs. 50, 51).

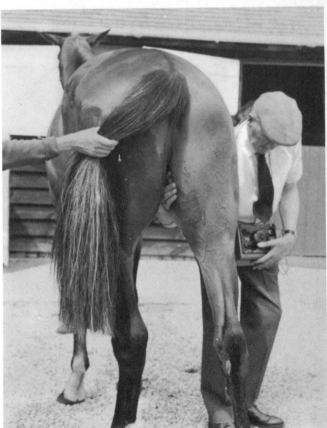

Fig. 48. By reaching well back on the inner side on the thigh the hindmost part of gracilis, adductor femoris and semi-membranosis can be treated

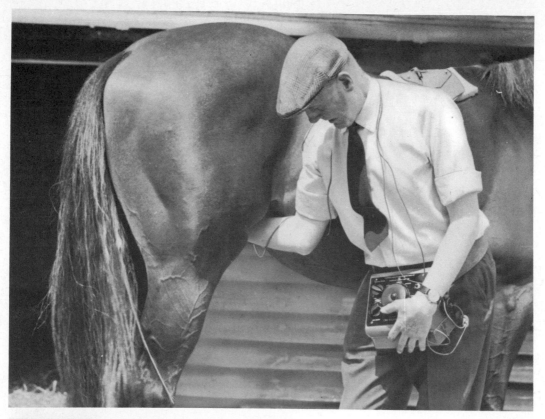

Fig. 49. Treating adductor muscles of Rt. thigh

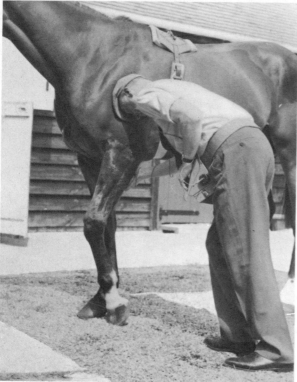

Fig. 50. If by pushing the horse's weight towards the opposite side, the animal will allow the leg under treatment to rest on the toe, thereby, gaining more effective treatment

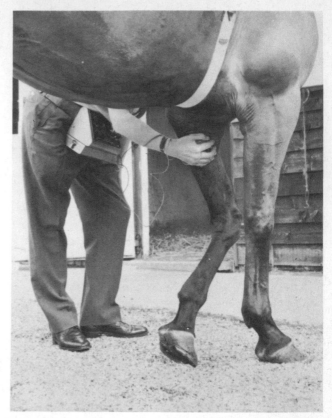

Fig. 51. Mobile electrode being applied to the flexor muscles of the Lt. forearm when treating the knee and all injuries below this level

Fig. 52. Although doing no harm, to apply the electrical current to the ringed areas will cause acute discomfort. There are no motor points here; to do so will achieve nothing

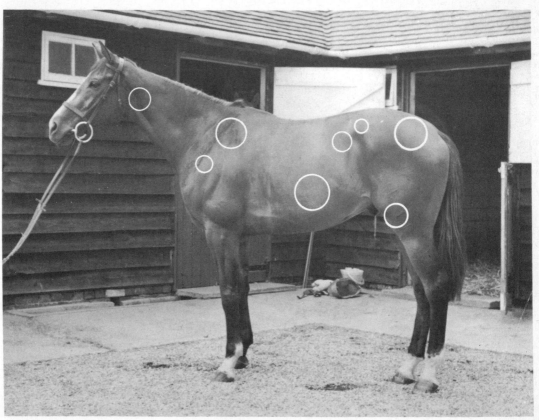

Notes on treatment to various regions

Areas normally hyper-sensitive to the electrical current and therefore to be avoided during treatment or investigation

All bony prominences and the areas ringed in Fig. 52.

When dogs are to be treated a special small roller is required (See Fig. 53)

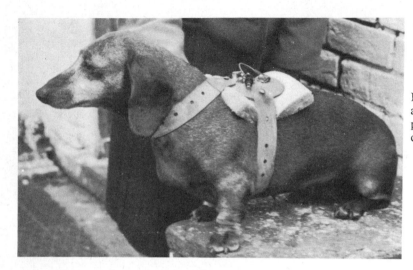

Fig. 53. A small roller and indifferent electrode pad are required when dogs are being treated

The author has treated a large number of horses of all types, the vast majority being 'flat' and 'N.H.' racehorses. Records show that cures are obtained in well over 80 per cent. of cases. Many of the racehorses have gone on afterwards to win many races and some even within days of the completion of treatment.

Of latter years horses under treatment have been in the care of Mr. Roger Stack, of Forest Green, Dorking, Surrey, England, to whom is owed a great debt of gratitude for the meticulous manner in which he has carried out instructions relative to exercise, an essential part of the treatment, including fast work, before the horses are returned home, and for producing the animals in such excellent 'condition' at this stage.

The possession of this apparatus is not an infallible indication of ability to use it efficiently.

Unless the operator is prepared to master the technique of diagnosis and the techniques of treatment of both fresh and old injury, to have determination with sensibility and patience to the utmost, to have the faithful co-operation of those responsible for the conduct of the prescribed exercise it is better he did not use the apparatus at all, as many brilliant and gratifying cures will elude him and so bring the method into disrepute.

Not as one new owner of this apparatus said after using it for ten minutes '. . . You are far too busy to deal with the work in this district, do tell everyone that I am the expert now . . .'

Index

Index

Index